HOW NOT TO GET FAT

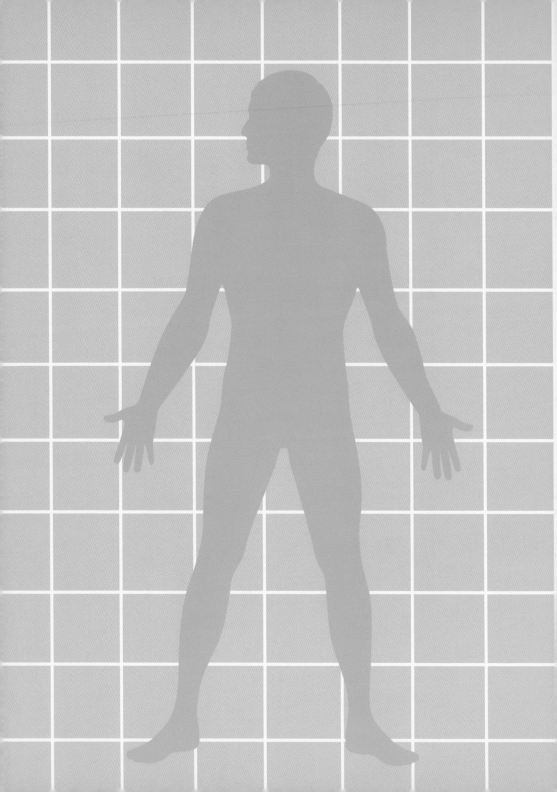

HOW NOT TO GET FAT

IAN MARBER

FIREFLY BOOKS

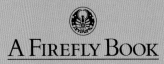

A FIREFLY BOOK

Published by Firefly Books Ltd. 2010

Text copyright © 2010 Ian Marber
Illustrations copyright © 2010 Lucy Vigrass

First printing

Publisher Cataloging-in-Publication Data (U.S.)

Marber, Ian.
    How not to get fat / Ian Marber, the Food Doctor.
[176] p. : col. ill.. ; cm
Includes index.
Summary: A practical and humorous guide that shows what to eat and when in order to maintain a healthy weight. Explains how the body works, how we think about food and dieting, and provides guidelines on good nutrition.
ISBN-13: 978-1-55407-775-5
ISBN-10: 1-55407-775-3
1. Diet therapy. 2. Nutrition. 3. Reducing diets. I. Title.
613.25 dc22 RM216.M373 2010

Library and Archives Canada Cataloguing in Publication

Marber, Ian.
    How not to get fat / Ian Marber.
ISBN-13: 978-1-55407-775-5
ISBN-10: 1-55407-775-3
1. Nutrition. 2. Health. I. Title.
RA784.M352 2010 613.2 C2010-903258-6

Published in the United States by
Firefly Books (U.S.) Inc.
P.O. Box 1338, Ellicott Station
Buffalo, New York 14205

Published in Canada by
Firefly Books Ltd.
66 Leek Crescent
Richmond Hill, Ontario L4B 1H1

Printed in China

How Not to Get Fat was developed by:
Quadrille Publishing Limited
Alhambra House
27-31 Charing Cross Road
London WC2H 0LS

Editorial Director Jane O'Shea
Creative Director Helen Lewis
Editor Susannah Steel
Designer Jim Smith
Illustrations Lucy Vigrass
Production Vincent Smith, Ruth Deary

Contents

Introduction

When I embarked upon the course that would lead to my career as a nutrition consultant, I was excited to be learning more about the potential of good nutrition and its effects on our health. Having already heard every cliché and quotation about food and nutrition—ranging from "You are what you eat" (an American proverb) to "Let food be thy medicine" (Hippocrates)—I had no doubt in my mind that an improved diet could have profound benefits, and I was delighted to have the opportunity to study again at the age of 32. During the first few months of studying my course, I even bored my friends and family with my newly acquired knowledge and gave many suggestions about which foods they should be eating.

However, I used to get quite irritated when people I met, when they learned I was studying nutrition, said something like, "Oh good, you can help me to lose some weight." I was studying serious, proper nutrition and was going to save the world from unnecessary illnesses; people were going to live longer, richer lives because of the improved nutritional advice they were going to receive from me. I wasn't going to go down the populist route and focus only on weight loss, and I instinctively resisted the shallow glory of helping people who were desperate to lose weight or who were fed up with dieting.

Once I had qualified as a nutrition consultant and started seeing clients, my heart would sink when I was asked for my advice on how to lose weight, as I really wanted to be talking about the serious stuff. I have to confess that weight loss quickly became my least favorite subject. I found that clients who wanted to lose weight were quite different from those who were seeking advice about, say, digestive issues or bloating, as they had usually already tried several diets and had valid reasons for why they failed. Although I gave advice that worked, it was an aspect of nutrition that I repeatedly wanted to shy away from.

The health and beauty director of a famous international glossy magazine asked me what the secret was for staying slim for life. My answer was simple: learn how to avoid putting on weight in the first place.

Looking back on this period now, I know that my reluctance to advise on weight issues was because I had nothing new to add to the debate. It wasn't until early in 2002 that I hit upon a practical and almost foolproof method for weight loss, much of which was covered in *The Food Doctor Diet* book series, first published in 2004. I remember that at the first book launch, a dear friend, who is, coincidentally, the health and beauty director of a famous international glossy magazine, asked me what the secret was for staying slim for life. My answer was simple: learn how to avoid putting on weight in the first place. They were easy words to say, and on the surface it seems such an obvious solution. Yet most people never expect or intend to put on weight, and as long as they remain slim they are unlikely to seek the advice of a nutrition consultant to help them learn how to avoid a potentially lifelong problem.

Every now and again you may hear an item in the news about an unusually large baby being born, or you may see an overweight child in a school playground, but they are in the minority; overweight, fat, plump, chubby, or heavy people rarely start out this way. So where are all the large people coming from? We certainly see more of them than we might have done 20 years ago. For example, in Britain, where I live, 46 percent of the adult male population and 32 percent of adult females are now overweight. An additional 17 percent of men and 21 percent of women are classified as obese. In the United States, the situation is even worse: according to the *Journal of the American Medical Association*, 32 percent of American men and 36 percent of women are obese. If we assume that a percentage of these overweight or obese people have become so through illness, incapacity, or injury, this still leaves a vast number of people who have become overweight or fat through years of improper eating and lack of exercise.

Overweight, fat, plump, chubby, or heavy people rarely start out that way. So where are all the large people coming from?

I am assuming—quite fairly, I think—that the majority of these people would choose not to have weight issues, and that circumstances have led them there. There are countless reasons why people might be overweight, but in my experience, ignorance is the most likely explanation. By this I mean simply that the reason why most people gain weight is that they don't fully understand how to eat in order to benefit their health and weight. Ask yourself this question: When were you taught how to eat in order to maintain a healthy weight? Few people can actually answer that question, in spite of it being a basic skill that each of us needs to know. I have heard it said many times that we should all be taught properly how to look after ourselves—life skills, if you like. So surely one of the most important of those skills is to know how to eat healthily. Bear in mind that the majority of the information we receive about the food we eat comes directly from the people who sell it to us (this is not to imply any conspiracy), and might not they have a vested interest in our food choices?

Ask yourself this question: When were you taught how to eat in order to maintain a healthy weight?

During my years in practice I have conducted several talks and workshops in schools, and I am always interested to see how much the children actually know about food and what they should eat. While I am not suggesting that we give young children lessons solely in staying trim, I wonder at what age or stage of education you would like to have been taught about how to eat for good health and weight management. Although we know that nothing in life is guaranteed, none of us really believe deep down that anything detrimental is going to happen to us; it's part of the human condition to feel immune to the events of life. I wonder if the vast number of people who are now classified as overweight could have imagined when they were younger that their fate would include weight problems, or even obesity, and whether being educated about how to eat properly would have meant a different future for them.

My fascination with educating people about good nutrition was sparked not just because I was consulted all the time about weight loss, but mainly because so many of the people who needed or wanted to lose weight were desperate to do so. Even clients in their 20s were battling with their weight, and had been on a diet of sorts since they were teenagers. The older my clients, the longer their stories. These stories were all different, but there was a shared feeling of frustration, much of which, I maintain, has been made worse by the confusion surrounding different diet plans.

Clients in their 20s were battling with their weight, and had been on a diet of sorts since they were teenagers; the older my clients, the longer their stories.

If we think about the most popular diets over the last 20 to 30 years, the ones that immediately spring to mind are:
- calorie controlled
- high fiber
- high protein
- low fat
- soup

No doubt you may be able to think of some others.

All these and other diets work to some extent simply because they limit the amount of food we eat by adding some rules and a framework for a certain period of time. If you follow a high-protein diet, for example, you have fewer choices and less room to make mistakes, and so the diet is easier to follow than your usual routine. The same could be said of any diet plan. Surely we could follow any one of these diets, lose the weight, and that would be that? It seems not, but why is this so? What's the problem?

Sadly, *we* are the problem.

When we finish a diet we tend to indulge ourselves, which is a direct result of having been restricted by the diet and guarantees a reason to have to go on another diet and be restricted again about what we can eat. Countless dieters have explained this dichotomy to me as they try to balance their food intake with one eye on living in the moment and enjoying life, and the other on being sensible.

Surely we could follow any diet, lose the weight, and that would be that? It seems not, but why is this so? What's the problem?

Over the years, I have identified an interesting link between how we manage our finances and the way in which we manage our weight, and you will see that I often use this analogy in this book to highlight points and to make matters clearer. For example, gaining weight, then losing it, and then repeating the cycle is akin to borrowing money to clear high-interest debts, as on credit cards, only to run them up to the credit limit again, leaving you with the card debt and the original loan to service. I have found that using this comparison of money and financial matters with clients makes it easier to talk about weight issues. It's clear to see that someone who is in turmoil over their finances—incurring debt and then borrowing money to clear it, time and time again—needs a guiding hand and some discipline. Yet when it comes to managing our weight, we seem happy to go it alone. What we weigh is as personal and as private as our finances should be, but carrying additional weight is, for many people, a physical sign that they are out of control in some way. For them, being overweight is a sign of failure and a source of shame.

Someone who is in turmoil over their finances needs a guiding hand and some discipline. Yet when it comes to managing our weight, we seem happy to go it alone.

What many of us don't realize is that the body works in a mechanical and dispassionate way when it comes to food. It extracts nutrients from what we eat and provides a supply of glucose to the body's cells, which then create energy. In order to lose weight, the body has to be managed and manipulated in a way that doesn't make it sense a major change in energy input or output, or "oncoming famine," which is effectively what a diet imposes. So our desire to want to lose weight quickly for an upcoming event such as a family wedding or a summer vacation does not marry well with the consistent requirements of our bodies. Nor do the mechanics of the body allow for prolonged periods of indulgence, such as December festivities, without having to make adjustments; our bodies are not interested in whether we plan to be "good" again after the weekend, or lose all the excess weight we put on in the previous month or year.

So *How Not to get Fat* is about learning to eat properly. We will be looking more closely at how our bodies work, exploring how our emotional thought processes and actions are usually at odds with this simple biochemistry, and finding out how to eat well without putting on weight. Experience tells me that most people would like to eat in a way that satisfies their hunger, allows them to eat good food, minimizes any cravings for particular foods, and is easily managed even with the busiest work schedule or social life—all without gaining weight. I believe that this book will show you clearly how to eat in a way that covers all these points and actually works, whether you need to lose weight or you are keen not to become fat in the first place.

Ian Marber
THE FOOD DOCTOR

SECTION ONE
HOW WE WORK

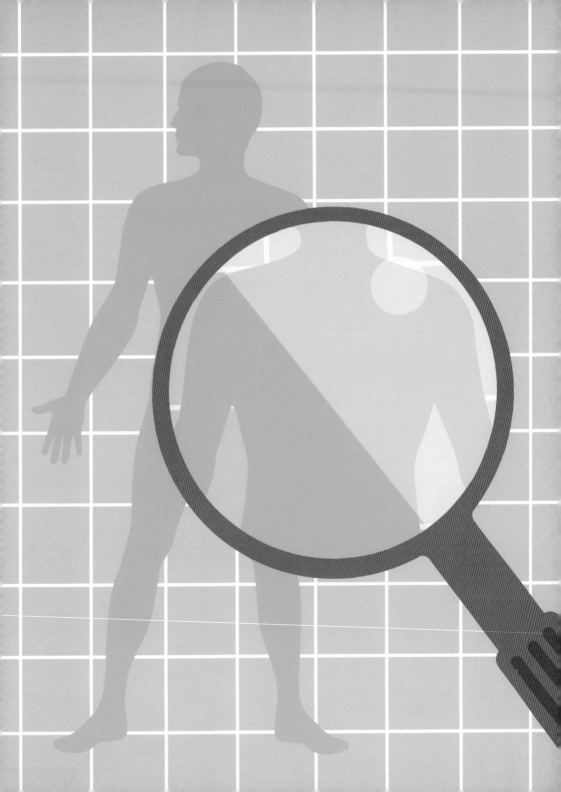

How our bodies work

In this first section we'll be looking at how the body works in relation to food and energy production. It is important that we understand some rudimentary facts about topics such as glucose, energy, metabolism, and the workings of the body, as they help to build the foundations of our knowledge about food and what we should eat. I don't know about you, but I didn't cover much biochemistry at school, and what was in the curriculum didn't help me learn how to eat, since I didn't make the connection. It wasn't until I returned to further education to study nutrition that biochemistry made any sense to me whatsoever.

The topics that we will cover here are those that I think we really need to understand.

I am not claiming the most in-depth knowledge of all aspects of this intricate subject, but I have been studying specific areas of it for almost 15 years now, and the topics that we will cover here are those that I think we really need to understand. We will pass over some topics quite rapidly and linger over others, and I have filtered out the unnecessary parts to simplify matters. Purists may feel that some of this explanation is simplistic, but I firmly believe that the reason why we become fat is not because we are lazy and greedy, but because we don't have an understanding of simple science. I know from lengthy experience that once we know how to eat, we can become immune to the misinformation that surrounds food and dieting. When I work with individual clients or large groups who grasp the basic tenet of how the human body absorbs the energy derived from what we eat and drink, they learn how to conquer weight gain once and for all.

"I never really understood the process of how fat was made until Ian drew it for me."
H. T

"After Ian explained it, it seemed obvious."
J. K.

How does food become energy?

Human beings eat primarily for one reason: survival. In order to survive, the body requires energy. Our digestive systems have evolved to extract energy from plants and other animals and distribute it to cells in the body that use it as fuel to create this necessary energy. Needless to say, this is an astoundingly detailed process, and one that is purely physiological: what we think or feel has little bearing on what occurs to our food once we have eaten it.

Biochemistry—the study of chemical processes that occur within us and other living organisms—is a highly intricate and complicated subject. The countless processes involved are so complicated that you would probably need a Ph.D. to understand them all fully. By the time I qualified as a nutrition consultant in 1999, my challenge was to find a reliable and foolproof way to communicate this knowledge to my clients, who had not had the luxury of three years of studying. Since then, I have worked on explaining the method by which glucose is extracted from food. For our purposes, we need to have a basic grasp of this process and how glucose is turned into energy. As it is imperative that we understand the main elements, allow me to give you a small taster of the basics we will explore in this section:

Glucose A simple sugar derived from food that is converted by the body into an important source of energy.

1 Food gets broken down into its constituent parts in the body, and glucose is extracted.
2 The glucose circulates in the blood.
3 Cells absorb the glucose and use it to make energy.
4 Any excess glucose that can't be absorbed is first stored in a water base in the muscles and liver and then converted into fat for longer-term storage.

In a nutshell, these are the headlines of what we need to know about glucose and energy, but we will delve into this more thoroughly over the coming pages.

Digestion

The process of digestion starts in the mouth with chewing. We know instinctively that we have to chew food in order to break it down, and in the mouth the bonds that hold food together gradually succumb to the action of our teeth and saliva. Although saliva is 99 percent water, it does contain digestive enzymes (notably lipase and amylase) in a weak state, which work on fats and carbohydrates respectively. The food is lubricated with saliva while it is being chewed, and once it has been broken down into a smaller lump or mass, known as a bolus, we then swallow it.

Digestion The process of breaking down food by mechanical and enzymatic action into substances that can be used by the body.

Enzyme A substance that speeds up the chemical changes in a living body.

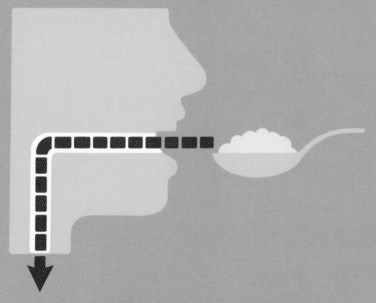

Passing through the throat, the food drops into the stomach, where it is bathed in various liquids that are secreted from cells located all around the internal lining of the stomach. These include gastric lipase, pepsin, and hydrochloric acid (HCl), the latter being the most abundant. The liquids wash over the food in waves, which are stimulated by involuntary muscle movement. They are gentle at first, but can become stronger the longer the food stays in the stomach. Little by little, as the various enzymes and acids infiltrate the food, it is reduced to a thin liquid called chyme.

Hydrochloric acid A strongly acidic solution of the gas hydrogen chloride in water.

Fiber The cell walls of plant foods. Fiber cannot be completely broken down by digestive enzymes in the body, but may be partly digested by bacteria in the intestine.

As long as the food remains in the stomach, it triggers the release of three hormones that we need to be aware of: gastric inhibitory peptide (GIP), cholecystokinin (CCK), and secretin. We don't need to look at everything these hormones do, but what we do need to know is that together they can slow down the rate at which the hydrochloric acid and other liquids wash over the food and break it down. Essentially this means that they help to make the food remain in the stomach for longer.

Not all food is broken down at the same speed. Carbohydrates spend the least amount of time in the stomach, proteins spend more time, and fats still more. The time they spend in the stomach relates to the physical make-up of the food itself, so if the food is thick and fibrous to chew, it will take a while for the hydrochloric acid and other substances to break it down. Conversely, if the food is easy to break down in the mouth, it will pass through the stomach quite rapidly; foods that are low in fiber or protein and contain little fat are typical examples of this type of food. We will look more closely at different foods in section three (pp.138–63), but at this stage all that is important for you to note is that not all food groups are created equal.

The stomach doesn't empty all at once, but empties in response to different reflexes one could consider unremarkable, at least for our purposes. However, the stomach can empty too quickly if the stomach is over-full, and also if alcohol or caffeine is present (this is a crucial element of digestion that we will pick up again in section three). The stomach also empties too quickly if it contains proteins that are partially undigested, which can occur when we don't chew our food properly or if the levels of stomach acid are low (good levels are needed to help break down all food, especially proteins).

Pancreas A large gland behind the stomach that secretes digestive enzymes into the intestine. Embedded in the pancreas are groups of pancreatic cells that secrete the hormones insulin and glucagon into the blood.

The stomach empties the liquid food into the duodenum, which is the highest part of the gastrointestinal tract. At this point we need to be aware of the role of the pancreas. This organ produces pancreatic liquid, which contains several enzymes that further break down fats, proteins, and carbohydrates. It is secreted into the intestine close to where the stomach empties the food so that it can be ready to work on the various elements. Once the food has entered the gastrointestinal tract, the process of absorption can really begin.

Why eat?

It is worth highlighting again that the point of eating is to provide energy, and glucose is the currency by which this energy is distributed to various cells in the body once it has been extracted from food. So the process of digestion is essential to enable the nutrients and glucose present in food to be made available to the body.

To recap, the stomach empties more quickly when it contains any of the following: alcohol, caffeine, or partially undigested protein. It also empties more quickly when it is over-full. However, the rate at which the stomach empties can be slowed down if the intestines instead are expanded with food.

The food is further diluted with intestinal juices and propelled toward finger-like protrusions called villi, which make up the site of absorption. What is important to know is that when the large intestine is swollen with food, a message is sent to the stomach telling it to slow down, which inhibits the process of digestion.

Villi Numerous minute elongated projections that extend the surface area of the lining of the small intestines and absorb nutrients into the bloodstream.

So the first part of the equation of how food becomes energy looks like this:

FOOD ▶ ▶ ▶ GLUCOSE

How does glucose enter cells?

For our purposes, it is glucose that is of prime importance in the process of absorption. Glucose is a simple sugar that is absorbed by the cells and used as fuel to make energy. Manipulating the levels of glucose available to your body is key to managing your energy levels, and therefore your weight. The simple explanation of this highly complex process is that glucose circulates around the body in the blood, ready to be absorbed by the cells in order to make energy.

So we can add another step to the equation:

FOOD ▶ ▶ ▶ GLUCOSE ▶ ▶ ▶ CIRCULATES IN BLOOD

These cells are sealed units, so the glucose doesn't arrive at a cell and just enter it. It has to be carried in, and only after the cell has been alerted to the presence of increased glucose levels in the blood.

Every cell is surrounded by a membrane, which acts much as skin does, providing a barrier to keep what is inside the cell where it should be and protect the cell from whatever is on the outside. In order for glucose to enter the cell, it has to be carried in on a transport protein (don't worry about the protein part of this description; it is simply the correct term for something that transports the glucose into the cell). I know this might sound too scientific, so take a look at the diagram of a cell below and see how the glucose surrounds it.

Insulin A hormone produced by the pancreas that circulates in the bloodstream and enables glucose to enter the body's cells. Insulin regulates the amount of glucose in the blood and converts excess glucose into glycogen and then fat to be stored in body tissues. Lack of insulin causes diabetes.

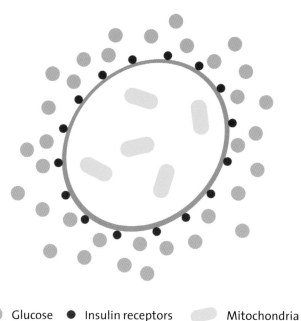

    ● Glucose   ● Insulin receptors   ● Mitochondria

This is only one side of the story, though, because the cell actually has to open up to allow the carrier—the transport protein—to enter. Around the image of the cell you will see little red dots, which are known as receptor sites. These receptor sites are sensitive to the presence of insulin, a substance that is also secreted by the pancreas. Insulin has several roles, but there are two that are most relevant:

First role

Insulin encourages the transport of glucose into the cells. The receptor sites register when insulin levels are rising, and instruct the cell to allow more glucose in.

Second role

Insulin encourages the conversion of glucose into glycogen, a temporary form of storage for excess glucose, which is held in the muscles and liver. When the glycogen stores in the muscles and liver become full, any more excess glucose is stored as fat.

Glycogen A form of excess glucose that is stored in the liver and muscles.

So our equation builds further:

FOOD ▸ ▸ ▸ GLUCOSE ▸ ▸ ▸ CIRCULATES IN BLOOD ▸ ▸ ▸ SURROUNDS AND ENTERS CELLS (WITH THE HELP OF INSULIN)

Insulin

Insulin is part friend and part foe when it comes to weight issues. Obviously, we need it in order to enable glucose to enter into the cells to make energy, but if we have too much glucose circulating in the blood, insulin will sweep away what it views as excess to our requirements and store it, rather than leaving it in the blood for the cell to use when it is ready. We can't actually store much glucose in its short-term state (as glycogen), so eventually the glucose is stored as fat in either existing or newly created fat cells.

Another substance, glucagon, is also produced by the pancreas and does the opposite from insulin, inasmuch as it increases levels of glucose in the blood if they fall too low. However, because keeping glucose levels low is one of the keys to controlling your weight, we will keep our focus on insulin, and glucagon won't figure much here.

It's important to point out that insulin works in a mechanical way, and is uninvolved in your thought processes. It has no idea that you may be eating a hearty breakfast because you won't be able to eat again for a few hours. Nor does it care if you are eating more than usual because you are at a friend's birthday dinner. It just quietly does its job. Aside from weight issues, insulin can also contribute to an increased appetite. This is because when insulin grabs the excess glucose in the blood to store it as glycogen in the liver and muscles, your glucose levels can actually fall too rapidly. At this point, glucagon (the counterbalance to insulin) tries to convert glycogen back into glucose (it is like one big turnstile, with glucose being converted to glycogen and back again), but low levels of glucose also encourage signals to be sent to the brain that say,

"FEED ME"

So we return to the cells and the circulating glucose. The level of insulin in the blood is directly linked to that of glucose, which is always present to one degree or another. As we have discovered, the concentration of glucose in the blood is regulated by glucagon and insulin: when glucose levels are high, insulin levels will rise accordingly. Just to remind ourselves, insulin is necessary to instruct the cell to open up to allow the glucose in.

The cell is limited in just how much glucose it can absorb at once. If the food that you have eaten is still being broken down into glucose—and the chances are that it will be—the overall levels of glucose in the blood are being added to at the same time that the cells are trying to absorb the existing glucose circulating in the blood. Imagine an egg timer with sand running through the narrow channel that divides the upper and lower sections, yet the sand in the upper section is being added to at a greater rate than the channel is emptying it into the lower section.

Glycogen

As the glucose in the blood builds up, it is the second role of insulin that we need to become more aware of. This involves the conversion of glucose to glycogen. Insulin manages glucose in the blood by enabling it to move into cells, but what the cells can't manage to absorb is converted into glycogen, the short-term storage version of glucose. The glucose that is waiting for the glucose ahead of it to be taken into the cells is grabbed by insulin and redirected straight into short-term storage in the muscles, liver, and, to a lesser extent, in tissue as well. When this short-term storage has reached capacity, the excess is stored away as fat around the body. Our glycogen levels are limited, but they can be enhanced, or increased, with exercise, allowing for more glucose to be stored in the short term and thereby discouraging the buildup of fat.

I am sure you are already beginning to see that if we can regulate the rate at which the stomach empties, so that it doesn't empty too quickly, and regulate glucose levels in the blood, weight control becomes a very real possibility. How you go about all this might still be a little baffling, but when I bring all the elements together you will see that it is easier than you might think.

What happens to glucose in the cell?

Mitochondria
Organelles (organized or
specialized structures),
present in most cells, that
play an important role in
the production of energy.

We have looked at how food becomes glucose and how the glucose
is distributed for use or stored away. The next link in the chain occurs
when the glucose is in the cell.

Glucose acts much like gasoline, as it feeds the cell (the engine),
that creates the energy that is needed for our bodies to work
(or the car to be driven).

Within every cell are mitochondria (the yellow lozenge shapes in the
diagram on p.22). These are immensely complex structures, which
have more than one role. The number of mitochondria found in a cell
varies greatly, and while some cells have very few mitochondria,
others have as many as 2,000. What we need to know is that these
complex units act as engines, producing energy, and use glucose as
their fuel.

A cell that contains an average amount of mitochondria (which is
estimated to be around 500) will absorb a certain amount of glucose,
but a cell that contains many more of these tiny power plants will
demand more fuel, and thus absorb more glucose. This potentially
leaves less glucose circulating around the outside of the cell.

So a cell with increased levels of mitochondria requires more fuel
in much the same way that an engine with more cylinders requires
more gasoline to function. It is possible to encourage the creation
of more mitochondria in the cells, which leads to greater amounts
of glucose being used and leaving less to be stored away.

White cells and brown cells

Although all cells are active to one degree or another, it would be fair to say that some are very active, while others are far less so. The active cells tend to be located in our muscles, and if we were to look at one under a powerful microscope it would seem dense, perhaps dark in color. This is due to the concentration of mitochondria that have multiplied in order to meet energy requirements, and which makes the cell likely to take in more glucose. By now you will realize that this means that less glucose is left to be stored away, so a highly active cell rather than an inactive cell is what we want. We often refer to these very active cells as being brown simply because they look dark in color when magnified. An inactive cell has fewer mitochondria and is paler, and is therefore referred to as a white cell.

To sum up, the completed equation looks like this:

FOOD ▶ ▶ ▶ GLUCOSE ▶ ▶ ▶ CIRCULATES IN BLOOD ▶ ▶ ▶ SURROUNDS AND ENTERS CELLS ▶ ▶ ▶ FUEL TO MAKE ENERGY

(BUT ANY EXCESS GLUCOSE THAT THE CELL
CANNOT ABSORB IS SWEPT AWAY FOR STORAGE.)

I hope you now understand that keeping blood-glucose levels steady is an essential part of weight control. However, this is not the whole story of how our bodies work, for the types of food we eat and how often we eat them are just as important to consider. We will look more closely at both of these areas on the following pages.

How foods affect glucose levels

Over the next few pages, we will look at various food groups and the way they differ in terms of how the body digests them. This is an important part of what we need to know about weight management, and, as before, I will be picking out only those aspects about each food group that I feel are most relevant and that will contribute further to developing a really easy and practical understanding of how our bodies work.

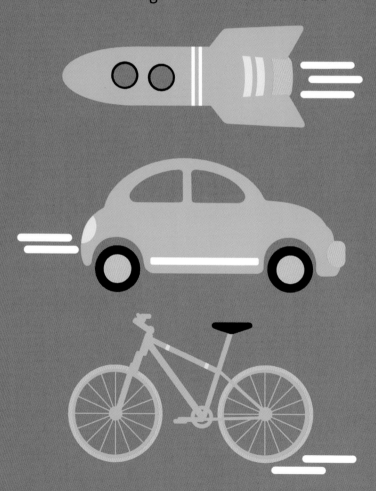

The three food groups

All foods are divided into three different food groups: carbohydrates, proteins, and fats. The speed at which they are broken down by the digestive system varies enormously. The rule of thumb is that carbohydrates (represented here by a rocket) are broken down most rapidly by the digestive system, proteins (symbolized by a car) are broken down more slowly, and fats (like a bicycle) are broken down slowest of all.

"Carbohydrates need to be managed carefully because they are potentially explosive foods."

"Proteins are dealt with in a more orderly fashion."

"Fat shouldn't be treated as if it were a four-letter word, but it needs to be regulated because of its high calorie content."

Carbohydrates

Carbohydrate A food derived from plant sources that contains sugars, starch, and fiber. It can be converted into glucose more readily than protein or fat. Carbohydrates can be classified as simple (containing little or no fiber) and complex (high in fiber).

Glucose is the body's preferred source of energy, and carbohydrates are the primary source of glucose. Carbohydrates are divided into two groups, simple and complex, and are made from a chain of sugars that are joined together (the chains can be of varying lengths). Carbohydrate foods are relatively cheap to grow, process, and store, which has partially contributed to their popularity.

Carbohydrates are the primary source of glucose.

Simple carbohydrates

This subgroup contains a short chain of sugars, which means that their physical form is effectively quite weak. The process of digestion described on pages 19–21 can deal easily with these simple sugars and break them down quickly. What this essentially means is that the glucose they contain can be extracted rapidly. No doubt you have heard of the glycemic index (or GI), which is a list of foods graded by the speed at which their glucose can be derived. The foods that give up their glucose the fastest are those at the upper end of the scale, and they are almost invariably simple carbohydrates.

Glycemic index A list that ranks foods on how quickly they break down in the body and affect blood-glucose levels. The foods are rated on a scale of 1 (low GI) to 100 (high GI).

Simple carbohydrates are very common in a Western diet and can be found in both natural and processed foods. For example, milk is a simple carbohydrate and so are most processed foods such as cake and cookies. Foods made from white flour also have a high score on the scale. Simple carbohydrates will generally contain a little fiber.

Ten simple carbohydrates

- Sugar
- Jam
- Pasta made from white flour
- Cake
- Cookies
- White bread
- Dried fruit
- Cereals (most)
- Fruit juice
- Milk

1 gram of simple carbohydrate is just under 4 calories.

Complex carbohydrates

These are made from a longer chain of sugars than contained in simple carbohydrates, and the digestive system takes longer to break them down into glucose. Therefore, the levels of glucose in the blood rise more slowly after a complex carbohydrate has been eaten. Complex carbohydrates contain more fiber than their simple counterparts.

The digestive system takes longer to break complex carbohydrates down into glucose.

Ten complex carbohydrates

- Beans
- Firm fruit
- Grapefruit
- Brown rice
- Rye
- Oats
- Green vegetables
- Brown bread
- Pasta made from whole wheat flour
- Barley

1 gram of complex carbohydrate contains about 4 calories.

An easy way to compare a simple carbohydrate and a complex carbohydrate is to think of simple carbohydrates as soft and complex carbohydrates as firmer. For example, compare a soft fruit such as a melon to a crisp apple. While they both contain fructose (fruit sugar), the digestive system will break down the melon far quicker than it will an apple, simply because the latter is dense and fibrous.

Which carbohydrate is better?

Both simple carbohydrates and complex carbohydrates serve a purpose, but because complex carbohydrates break down more slowly in the body, their effect on blood-glucose and insulin levels is gradual, rather than pronounced. It would be fair to say that, for our purposes, complex carbohydrates are better than simple carbohydrates although, once again, that's not the whole story.

Proteins

Protein A food derived from either animal or plant that is broken down by the body into amino acids, which are essential for the growth of cells and tissue repair.

Proteins are a combination of amino acids that are held together by links known as peptide bonds. In this context we don't need to look closely at amino acids (either their numbers or ideal combinations) or peptide bonds, as those are the kind of details that muddy the waters. Nor do we need to go into detail about what proteins do. What is important to note is that proteins are broken down by the process of digestion and are used all over the body, especially in the physical structure of muscles and tissue.

Protein is found mostly in animals, so the flesh of any animal will provide dietary protein. If you imagine chewing a piece of chicken breast or steak (not all proteins come from animals; there are a few sourced from vegetarian foods as well), you will have an idea of how hard it is to break down protein. Its physical structure is very dense, and it takes the strong nature of hydrochloric acid in the stomach to start working on separating the peptide bonds that hold the protein together. It is not until these bonds are loosened and separated that the protein is in a suitable form to be passed into the intestine.

Protein is not directly used to make glucose. Instead, it releases its amino acids, which contribute to the process of making energy through another substance (called pyruvic acid). If carbohydrates are limited in availability, the body can use protein to make energy.

The key importance to us in this context is the complex nature of protein, which results in a slow passage through the digestive system. So the breakdown of protein in comparison to that of explosive carbohydrates is slow.

Proteins

All meat, fish, and poultry are protein sources.

Plant proteins:

- Beans
- Hempseed nuts
- Nuts
- Seeds
- Soy (and products such as tofu)
- Quinoa

1 gram of protein contains around 4 calories.

Fats

Dietary fats are a type of lipid (compound) made from fatty acids and glycerol that are held together by bonds, which form a chain that makes them flexible. Some fats are liquid at room temperature, while others are solid, which reflects the density of the chains and their chemical makeup. For example, a fat such as olive oil has a flexible chain and so is viscous, while lard has a denser chain, which is why it is solid at room temperature. Like protein, most fats take a while to be worked on in the stomach.

Dietary fats do not break down in water and are not digested by the body until they have left the stomach and are broken down into fatty acids and glycerol. Fat is absorbed and transported around the body, but it is rarely used to make energy because glucose is the body's preferred source of fuel. Only glycerol can easily be used to make energy, but this constitutes only a small part of the fat that we eat. The rest of the fatty acids are either used in metabolic or structural processes or stored away in fat cells (although some is oxidized and made available as a source of energy). In simple terms, only a small amount of the fat we eat is used to make energy, especially if the body has an abundant source of glucose on hand.

When we eat fat, the hormones CCK and GIP (p.20), which are designed to send messages of feeling full to the brain, are released. Furthermore, in the mouth the process of eating anything containing fat provides what the food industry calls "mouthfeel," which enhances the experience of eating. Simply put, this enhances the feeling of satisfaction after having eaten fat.

Fat An oily component in plant and animal foods that contains fatty acids. It is a concentrated source of energy. Fats can be classified as saturated (often solid at room temperature and usually from animal sources) and unsaturated (usually liquid at room temperature and generally from plant sources).

Fats

- Nuts
- Seeds
- Fish
- Red meat
- Poultry
- Dairy products
- Oils (such as olive oil)

1 gram of fat contains 9 calories.

What else raises glucose levels?

What we eat is not the only thing that influences the concentration of glucose in the bloodstream. There are also several lifestyle factors that we should be aware of, since they, too, need to be managed (inasmuch as it is possible to manage them) if we are to maintain a healthy weight. In section three we will be looking at how we can manage these factors more effectively, but in this section we need to look a little more closely at how they affect the digestive process and what they do to raise blood glucose.

Does having raised glucose levels matter?

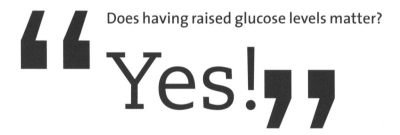

"Yes!"

As we have already discovered, glucose is always present in the blood, and its levels are regulated by glucagon and insulin. In terms of weight gain, raised levels of glucose encourage insulin to be released at the same time to regulate the glucose. When we do or eat things that encourage glucose levels to get too high, fat can be created. We know that insulin wants to enable glucose to enter the cell, but we also know that what the cell cannot absorb is going to be diverted by the insulin to be stored away as glycogen or fat.

Stress

I have an image of a "stressed" person, one that is very much prompted by popular perceptions (I apologize for the stereotypes). If I think of what a stressed man might look like, he would probably be dressed in a suit and tie, the tie would be pulled open a little, and he would be sitting at a desk that is strewn with paperwork, telephones, and a computer screen. A woman might be under the same pressure at her workplace, or perhaps at home surrounded by active children with shopping to unpack and meals to prepare.

These stereotypical images of what a stressed person might look like are, of course, entirely wrong, because the simple truth is that we all live with degrees of stress; what differs is how we handle it. We might seem capable and in charge on the outside, or we might be anxious and seemingly unable to cope.

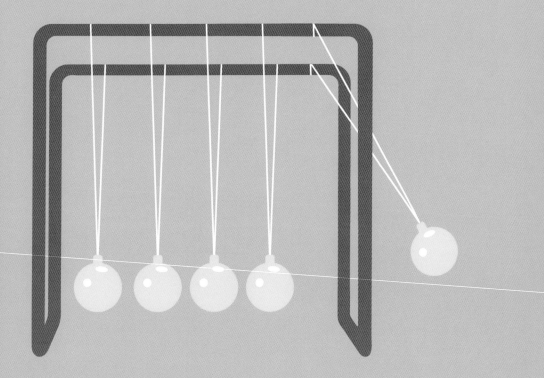

When it comes to stress as a factor that raises blood-glucose levels, it doesn't matter whether you fall into any of the stereotypes that I have described, what sex you are, or whether you work, study, or keep a home. Stress, in this context, is a physical reaction to an external stimulus. The biochemical reactions to stress that take place in the body occur whether we like it or not, and whether the reason for the stress is something that someone else might find quite trivial.

> The biochemical reactions to stress that take place in the body occur whether we like it or not, and whether the reason for the stress is something that someone else might find trivial.

For example, the physiological response to stress is the same for the person who is rushing to catch a bus loaded down by shopping and a young child as it is for someone worrying about whether inclement weather will prevent their private jet from landing at the airport nearest to one of their several luxurious homes. We might feel less sympathy for the jet owner, but stress still triggers a chain of biochemical reactions in spite of such relatively trivial worries.

When the body senses a threat of any kind, epinephrine (also called adrenaline) is produced by the adrenal glands in order to prepare the body for the situation. We developed this reaction to allow us to meet physical threats and situations, such as being attacked or hunting for food. For this reason the rush of epinephrine we experience when we are stressed is called the "fight or flight" response, as the body undergoes physical changes that prepare it either to fight or flee—both of which require increased levels of energy and alertness. I think it is fair to say that the modern age has few situations that are quite so threatening in a physical way, yet we now have to respond to various other forms of stress, which can be anything that makes you anxious or nervous. The epinephrine is released in just the same way as if we were about to be pounced upon by a predator, and because sources of stress are all around us and constant, adrenaline release is likely to increase accordingly.

Adrenaline has several effects on the body, the most relevant to us being its influence on blood glucose and hunger. In times of stress, glycogen (the temporary stored form of glucose) is broken down by epinephrine to offer a quick boost of glucose to meet the increased demand in energy. These days, this might be used for mental energy as much as physical energy, and as such is often in demand.

If you add this information to what we have already covered in the previous pages, you will know now that raised levels of glucose in the blood lead to an increase of insulin alongside it. This means that some of the excess glucose that was released will be recycled back into glycogen and stored temporarily, and then stored as fat.

Epinephrine A hormone secreted by the adrenal glands (and sometimes called adrenaline) in response to exercise, low blood-glucose levels, and stress. It increases blood circulation and breathing and prepares muscles for action by causing glycogen stores to be converted to glucose and fatty acids to be released from tissues to increase blood-glucose levels.

In times of stress, glycogen (the temporary stored form of glucose) is broken down by epinephrine to offer a quick boost of glucose to meet the increased demand in energy. These days, this might be used for mental energy as much as physical energy, and as such is often in demand.

Caffeine

As I mentioned on pages 20 and 21, caffeine encourages the stomach to empty its contents into the digestive system possibly faster than is ideal. This can then have an effect on the amount of glucose that is produced: under the influence of caffeine, food is processed faster than the body was designed for, which raises glucose levels.

Caffeine also triggers the release of epinephrine, and so works in a similar way to other sources of stress. Caffeinated drinks are often free of calories, which make them especially attractive to people who are following a low-fat diet. However, when we drink a cup of coffee or tea, a glass of cola, or any caffeinated soft drink, some of the caffeine

Under the influence of caffeine, food
is processed faster than the body was
designed for, which raises glucose levels.

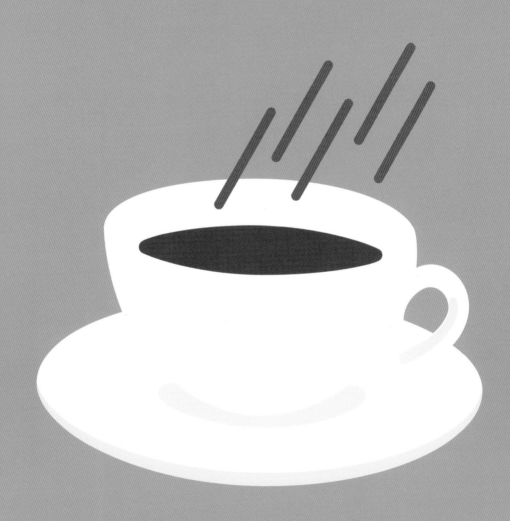

is absorbed in the stomach, which is why it is so fast-acting. The rest is absorbed in the intestine, so the effects are extended for a while. Once caffeine enters the bloodstream, it is taken to the brain, where it settles in receptor sites. These sites are designed to accept a different substance, adenosine (which, coincidentally, has the same shape—like a jigsaw piece), which actually works to calm the body, unlike caffeine. However, when caffeine occupies those same sites the brain is stimulated, rather than calmed, which the adrenal glands interpret as stress. They respond to this stimulation by releasing epinephrine, which compounds the situation.

Caffeine therefore influences the speed at which foods are processed in the stomach, and also raises glucose levels, which will in turn trigger increased levels of insulin. Caffeine in the diet comes from several sources. Obviously it's to be found in coffee, tea, and cola drinks, but it is also found in chocolate and other cocoa products.

Smoking

Nicotine has countless effects on the body, but in terms of weight issues, its effects are both physiological and psychological. Inhaling nicotine causes an increase in epinephrine and so acts much like stress in influencing glucose levels. Furthermore, nicotine masks the hunger response in the very short term, which helps quash appetite—albeit for a matter of minutes. Many people who smoke are anxious about giving it up, fearing what they believe will be inevitable weight gain.

The metabolic rate

Many people will cite a slow metabolism as the reason for their weight problems. Put simply, the metabolic rate is the number of calories that the body requires to maintain itself. Every function requires energy, from movement to thought and digestion to breathing. The primary source of the energy that we need to function well is what we eat and drink.

It's worth reminding ourselves once more that glucose is extracted from food and then circulates in the blood. When it enters cells, it is used to make energy. If our food intake increases, the glucose levels in the blood become too concentrated, and insulin signals for the excess glucose to be stored away, first as glycogen and then as fat. Conversely, if our food intake reduces, the body will dip into its reserves of fat, forcing them to be converted back into glucose to make up for the deficit.

When we increase our output of energy—either through increased general activity or through bursts of exercise—fat is once again broken down to allow glucose to be released back into the energy chain unless we increase our food intake accordingly.

These inputs and outputs (deposits and withdrawals, if you like) take place to some degree every day, and small deficits are unlikely to cause any changes to our metabolic rate. However, the more often we tax our systems by making radical changes (such as dieting), the more likely we are to influence the way that our metabolic system works.

How do dieting and exercise affect our metabolic rate?

We might decide, for example, that we want to be healthier, so we choose to adopt a rigorous exercise program and start dieting. There are countless reasons why we might do this, including weight gain, a milestone birthday, a family get-together, or illness. Whatever our reasoning for undertaking a change in lifestyle, and however sound it may seem to be, our bodies run as machines and are completely unaware and uninterested in the question "Why?" Instead, they respond to "How."

In the very short term, if you have overeaten for a couple of days and then rein back on your food intake, your metabolism may be alerted to the increase, but it is unlikely to alter its workings unless the situation continues for several days. The same is true when you are careful about what you eat while following a low-calorie diet. If your intake is a little lower, the fat that was once glucose will be broken down to create energy to make up for the deficit.

Metabolism The rate at which glucose is used up by body cells to create energy.

Our bodies run as machines and are unaware and uninterested in "Why?"

However, the human condition is such that we want to see results, and see them quickly. We want proof that our investment of time and energy is paying off, so the diet you choose tends to be dramatic and punitive. Even if you don't cut out too many calories, your increased exercise and activity create a noticeable difference between what you consume and the energy you expend. Your metabolic rate has no idea about your carefully constructed plans. Instead, it dips into its reserves: first glycogen, which is quickly depleted, and then fat, forcing the cells to give up their fat to allow it to be converted back into glucose.

Try thinking of glucose as money in a checking account, glycogen as a line of credit, and fat as a savings account. If you have a cut in salary, say, you know that you will have to budget. The same is true of your metabolism, as it allows the savings account to be cleared out to make sure that there is enough glucose to go around.

Try thinking of glucose as money in a checking account, glycogen as a line of credit, and fat as a savings account.

However, the problem lies not in the first diet, or even the second. It is when you habitually have a chaotic and inconsistent intake of food and output of energy that your metabolism becomes confused.

Back to the money analogy: Your bank manager sees you clear out your checking account, go through your overdraft, and then work your way through what you had in savings. When you have reached your target weight, and the three sessions a week at the gym seem too much like hard work, you ease off a little and stop trying so hard.

When you habitually have a chaotic and inconsistent intake of food and output of energy, your metabolism becomes confused.

Your metabolism has no idea that some goal has been reached, or that you are now too busy to continue with your exercise regime. All it sees is an increase in energy intake and a decrease in output. Your bank manager would see that you can't be trusted with money, as your spending and saving habits are erratic. While your bank manager may respectfully advise you that you should open a long-term savings account and put a set amount away to save for a rainy day, your body may do the equivalent without any of the niceties. It will store fat away, as you have alerted it to the likelihood of potential famine, and the fat that it stores away becomes increasingly difficult to break down, however hard you exercise and however stringently you try to diet.

If you keep dieting, the fat that your body stores away becomes increasingly difficult to break down, however hard you exercise and however stringently you diet.

Aging and the metabolic rate

It is a widely held belief that the metabolic rate slows down with age; and, indeed, it is a part of getting older. As a result, we will inevitably gain weight if we continue to enjoy a high intake of food. However, the rate at which the metabolism slows down is also directly related to how many times we have dieted and overeaten in the past, as well

How our metabolism can change for the worse

Some people are born with a naturally high metabolic rate whereas other people have a slower metabolism (which can be enhanced to some degree by exercise). However, the process of dieting, and especially that of repeated dieting, has a negative effect on even the fastest metabolism, as the body is programmed to sense potential famine and will work to reset itself to conserve energy for the future.

as the level of physical activity and exercise we continue—or not—to undertake. We tend to be less physical as we age, and so this could contribute to the reduction in energy requirements, which in turn slow down our metabolism.

FOOD ▸ ▸ ▸ GLUCOSE ▸ ▸ ▸ CIRCULATES IN BLOOD ▸ ▸ ▸ SURROUNDS AND ENTERS CELLS ▸ ▸ ▸ FUEL TO MAKE ENERGY
(BUT ANY EXCESS GLUCOSE THAT THE CELL CANNOT ABSORB IS SWEPT AWAY FOR STORAGE.)

Hopefully you can see how we now have a sound understanding of some potentially complicated biochemistry. Take a look at this last equation again, which summarizes all that we have covered in this first section. As you turn to section two, keep this information in mind and remember that the key to weight control lies in relating how we work to what we eat, not how we think or the careful diet plans that we make.

SECTION TWO
HOW WE THINK

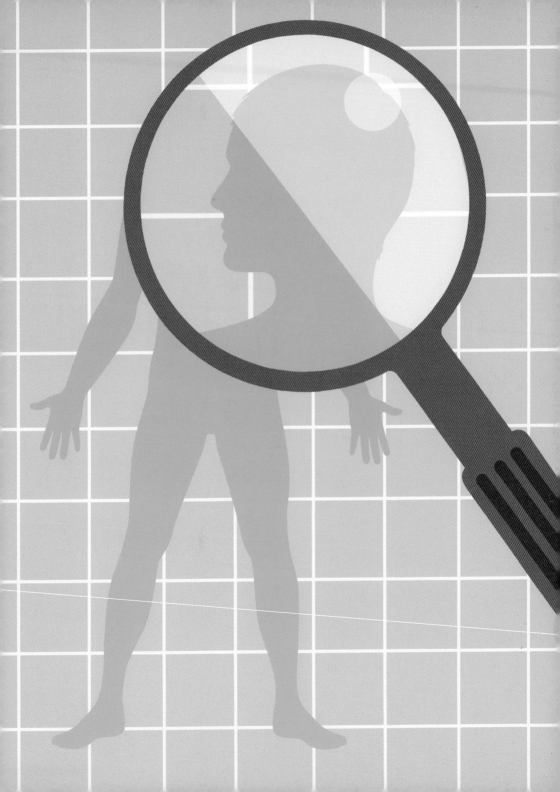

How our brains work

If you have dieted and regained the weight even once, worried about how much you weigh, chosen to eat low-calorie foods to control your weight, resisted certain foods in an effort to curb your appetite, or taken up exercise specifically to lose weight, then you are one of the vast majority of people who may spend much of their adult life on a diet of sorts.

Diets are the equivalent of riverside resuscitation stations, which tend to unlimited numbers of people who have half-drowned in their attempt to swim upstream without ever having been taught how to swim properly in the first place.

When you think about the diets that you might be familiar with, they are, with few exceptions, commercially driven. Whether they are run by a large multinational organization that holds regular meetings, based around the theory of a health professional, or fronted by a celebrity, there is money to be made. This doesn't mean that these diets aren't well intentioned, but in order to get you to buy into their program, they have a unique aspect that differentiates them from other diets. I remember reading about a diet, for example, that suggested we eat food that contained a specific type of essential fat. I am sure that if you followed this particular diet for a while you would lose some weight, but then, over time, put on the weight again. The same could be said about most diets.

I maintain that it is a combination of ignorance about how our bodies work and repeated attempts at dieting that are major factors in the almost global obesity epidemic we are experiencing now. I don't think we are taught how to eat appropriately in school, and what we learn about food and our weight comes mostly from advertising and the popular media. Diets dominate our magazines and newspapers, and stories of how a celebrity may have lost weight after going on a diet are headline news all over the world.

It is a combination of ignorance about how our bodies work and repeated attempts at dieting that are major factors in the almost global obesity epidemic we are experiencing now.

Diets are the equivalent of riverside resuscitation stations that tend to unlimited numbers of people who have half-drowned in their attempt to swim upstream without ever having been taught how to swim properly in the first place.

This leads to a major misconception about food, and we are paying the price in terms of our physical and emotional health. If you are unconvinced by this argument, you may want to find a photograph of yourself taken at a time when you thought you were fat. If you don't have a photo, ask an older friend or relative who has battled with their weight to dig one out. There is a very high chance that you will look at the photo of yourself and see someone who was a little overweight, but nowhere near as fat as you assumed you were. Yet the diet you undertook to get rid of that weight was inappropriate and too strict, which led to hunger and feelings of deprivation that triggered an emotional response from you to a purely physiological situation. Any subsequent actions you took would have been driven by this knee-jerk reaction, which probably led to initial weight loss followed by almost inevitable weight gain. Fast-forward a few years, and the weight you are battling with now is as much linked to how you dieted years ago as to what you ate last weekend.

We learn how to diet, not how to eat.

Attitudes and emotions

Being overweight means different things to different people. I find it unsettling when the word "fat" is used as an insult, yet fat people are teased and ridiculed in a way that would be unacceptable if they had different, yet equally evident, physical attributes. It is deemed socially acceptable to poke fun at fat people, which I imagine is because they are viewed as being entirely responsible for their current situation. If you are thinking, "Well, they are fat, aren't they?" then I have to ask, "What does being fat mean to you, and what do you think of fat people?" Take a moment and ask yourself how you really feel about fat people, and if you are, or have been, overweight, how you feel (or felt) about yourself. I would hope that most people who are overweight are kind to themselves, entirely aware of how it happened, and feel relaxed about eating and exercising in a way that will help to rid them of this excess weight over a sensible period of time. But while I am sure that there are many people who fall into this category, I am equally sure that there far more people who are not so kind to themselves. You may see your weight gain as a sign of moral failure, and you are embarrassed about your size. Even if your friends, family, or colleagues don't think you are especially fat, what they think doesn't count for much; we all know that it's what we think of ourselves that determines our behavior.

I certainly don't want to demonize overweight people or make any moral judgments in this book, nor do I have any personal feelings about other people's weight and whether they are fat or thin; their size does not influence my opinion of them. However, having conducted more than 5,000 one-to-one consultations, worked with participants on several television shows, and received countless e-mails and letters from people who struggle with their weight, I have witnessed the misery and shame that many people might feel when they are overweight. They feel unattractive, self-conscious, out of control, ashamed of themselves, and second-rate. They may avoid social situations, sexual or romantic encounters, and family events, due to embarrassment and fear of being judged. Finding clothes becomes increasingly difficult, as they may want to hide away and not be noticed. Even if their confidence has not been dented, finding clothes that make them look and feel good can be problematic, as clothes in larger sizes tend to be unfashionable. The list of social stigmas that go hand in hand with being fat is long, and if you relate to anything on this list, I am sure there are plenty of other situations and feelings you could add to it.

Having worked with so many clients over the years, I asked several of them to tell me how they felt when they were overweight. I am sure that the feelings of these individuals will be familiar to anyone who has struggled with their weight.

"I was ashamed of myself, but I found myself being that jolly fat person. I made jokes about myself before other people could."

H. T.

"I had lost weight and put it back on, but I kidded myself that I had got away with it as no one had said anything."

H. C.

"I felt that when anyone looked at me, all they saw was a fat person. My husband always said that he loved me 'no matter what,' but when I lost weight he became far more interested in me, not just physically. It was as if I had regained my place in the world when I was slimmer."

M. L.

How different are we really?

For those of you who are slim, and who are reading this book to ensure that you maintain a healthy weight, there is a chance that some of what you will read in this section may seem far-fetched. You, like other members of your family, may be naturally slim and have been physically active since a relatively young age. If this sounds familiar to you, then you may think that your chances of gaining weight are probably less than the majority of the population. You may read this section and think that such things happen to "other people" —but think again. Those "other people" were not born fat. Their weight has increased little by little as they have reacted to situations in life without the knowledge they needed to know in order to eat properly. If you are not fat, but you are dieting without a full understanding of the medium- and long-term cost of your chosen regime, you are on the same road, albeit not as far, as someone who is fat. (By "fat" I don't mean someone who is vast and has to have walls removed to leave their house, although they are simply farther along the same road as someone who is more than just a few pounds overweight.) It is my opinion that if we know how to eat in a way that is in harmony with how our bodies work, our weight will be far less of an issue than it is. In other words, if we know how to eat so that we are satisfied and don't feel hungry, we won't tamper with our metabolic rate by dieting, and any weight gain will be minimal.

This section exposes the claims and unfulfilled promises of diet programs and uncovers the confused feelings and mixed reactions we have toward food and the emotions we prefer to keep hidden about the issue of being overweight. If you are still unsure of the physiological reaction of our bodies to food, refresh your mind by looking again at the simplified equation on page 27 or page 43 of section one. Then begin this section feeling confident that you now know the essential facts about how our bodies work as we explore the issue of our weight and the misleading thought processes that we are so prone to.

This section exposes the claims and unfulfilled promises of diet programs and uncovers the confused feelings and mixed reactions we have toward food and the emotions we prefer to keep hidden about the issue of being overweight.

The issue of hunger

From a very early age, we know that being hungry is something that needs to be addressed. As young infants, our crying was a sign of hunger, and we were fed. Throughout our childhood, our parents would undoubtedly have asked if we were hungry and fed us accordingly. Hunger is an entirely normal feeling we experience when various hormones reach the brain, and it is something we should respond to. Yet as adults we often ignore the signal that tells us we are hungry. We know that we should eat, but since eating can be an anxious experience for many of us, this signal to eat can be confusing, if not alarming, so we choose to ignore it.

Why is this? What is wrong with being hungry, and why do so many people fear it? It may seem obvious, but I feel that most people think that if their hunger can be conquered, their eating can be controlled. In effect, food is seen as a battleground, and the signal to attack is hunger, so it's no wonder that food becomes something to be conquered. One could argue that this is all the wrong way around: if there are any issues with eating, then surely responding to the very first sign of hunger in an appropriate and measured way would help to avoid the battle with food altogether. But in practice, instead of responding to that hunger signal, people will often try to muddle through until the next scheduled meal and spend that interim period of time resisting temptation.

The emotion of hunger

If we look at the language associated with being hungry, "hunger" is most often followed by the word "pangs," which means "a sharp feeling or spasm of pain or emotional distress." If this is true—and it is for a large percentage of the population—then we might be able to see why the issue of hunger is such an emotional minefield.

The signal that your body sends you to refuel is triggered by several things, of which perhaps the most notable, as we discovered in section one, is low blood-glucose levels. In section three I will be explaining how to eat so that your blood-glucose levels can be maintained at an even level to avoid extreme and true hunger, but here we should explore what happens to the average weight-conscious person when they get that biochemical signal that says,

"FEED ME"

That signal to eat may come from a basic physiological need, and although our ancestors may have responded appropriately if food was available, these days our hunger is clouded by several issues, not least the thought of what we might weigh if we "give in" and eat something. Our emotional life gets in the way and greatly influences our decision.

"Being hungry was the gateway to hell for me. If I was on a diet, then all it did was make me obsess about what I couldn't eat."
J. H.

"I did everything I could to pretend I wasn't hungry. If I allowed myself to feel hungry, even if it was time to eat, then I had lost the battle that day. And when I lost the battle, I didn't stop eating; not that much, I suppose, but more than I wanted or needed."
C. C.

Ticker-tape thoughts

When our brain receives that signal from our body that food is required, we will either be motivated to get something to eat or resist that impulse. The sequence of contradictory thoughts played out here may be familiar to you …

I'm hungry

What's wrong with me? I've only just eaten. It's only three o'clock and I can still taste lunch …

I really shouldn't be hungry. I am sure that I read somewhere that I should eat little and often. But what does "little" mean? And "often," for that matter?

Well, I suppose I should eat something, but I don't want to get fat. I am being good at the moment. OK, so I'll have an apple. But I don't want an apple. Maybe I could have some raisins, that's still fruit, isn't it?

Why am I hungry? It's only an hour since lunch, I am sure I can hang on a little while, I am never going to lose weight if I eat all the time …

I could have a low-fat yogurt, or one of those granola bars I saw on television …

Hmmm… maybe I could go to the health-food store, it has healthful snacks, which can't be bad, can they?

I work really hard, for heaven's sake. I am too busy to worry about this, and anyway, he [she] loves me whatever size I am.

Anyway, who cares what I eat? It shouldn't matter what I weigh. So what if I am a few pounds heavier than I used to be?

If I lose too much weight, I look skinny. *But I'm still hungry …*

I don't know why I concern myself about such shallow things …

The gateway to confusion

One of the problems with being hungry in the twenty-first century is the matter of choice. There is now so much choice that we don't know what or how to eat, and hunger is the gateway to all that potential confusion. If you aren't hungry, the struggle is minimized. One of the reasons why strict diets can be successful is that they remove all choice: when you feel hungry, you are told to eat X or Y, a prescribed food that feels "safe." There is no choice, no confusion, and no argument. The internal dichotomy ("Should I, shouldn't I?") simply doesn't exist; this whole area of conflict is removed and you are not held responsible. After you have finished a diet, or even if you have never been on one, there are unlimited food choices to distract, confuse, and overwhelm you, and given how much commercial interests influence what foods we think of, we may eat in a way that doesn't serve us well.

> "Eating out was always a problem as there was too much choice and I simply didn't trust myself."
>
> **S. K.**

It's like choosing a meal from a long menu: you are not quite sure what you want and so you peer around you to see what other customers have chosen to eat. After you have ordered, dishes destined for the other tables are carried past you and you are never quite happy with your choice. Compare this confusion to a set menu with three appetizers and three entrées to choose from, where the chances are that you will make your choices without second-guessing yourself. There's more discussion of this issue later on in section two (pp.82–87), but there's no doubt that the number of choices available to you when you are not on a diet can be overwhelming.

Refuel or run out of energy?

I always advise my clients to respond to their hunger and see it as an opportunity to refuel, rather than as a reminder of potential failure.

However, this is not an easy concept to take on board, and the cold-hearted mechanics of the hunger response can be demonstrated by comparing the human body to a car.

Imagine this: you are driving your car (if you don't own a car or don't drive, do read this, as I am confident that you will still relate to this clear analogy). You notice that the level of gas left in the tank is getting low. You can't quite remember when you last stopped for gas, but you are aware that you need to fill up soon. The warning light isn't on yet, though, so the requirement isn't too pressing. You are short of time, and you would prefer not to spend money on filling up with gas at the moment. But then the light on the dashboard flashes, informing you that the gas level is now very low.

Do you
A) Think about your planned route and destination and make a rational decision to stop off at a convenient gas station soon to fill up the car?
Or
B) Pull the car over to the side of the road to have a word with it? After all, you filled it just last week, and it's simply going to have to get by until the weekend when you have the time to fill up again. And that's all there is to it. No arguments.

Put like this, the answer is obvious, isn't it? You must factor in the time and expense of filling up the tank, and you do so. Answer A is the only choice. Your car is a machine that requires refueling, and so do we. The hunger signal in us is just like the gas warning light in the car, and we need to respond in the same logical, unemotional way by eating something that will sustain us until the next time we have to refuel. This doesn't mean you can't enjoy the foods you eat, but if you can master this basic principle, the hunger you experience can be enjoyed as a prelude to good food and sensible decisions rather than feared and fought against. I'll be explaining a simple way to do this in section three, after we've investigated more about our attitudes to food and eating.

Real hunger versus fraudulent hunger

There is nothing wrong with being hungry, yet I know from experience that many people fear this very basic and normal response. Genuine hunger results from a variety of biochemical signals that inform the brain that fuel is required. Hormones and neurotransmitters are released, which influence our appetite. However, these biochemical signals influence what could be termed "true hunger," which is the hunger we experience when the body requires glucose to keep functioning normally.

There are, of course, other reasons why we eat, and these often have nothing to do with real hunger. They include, but are not limited to, the following.

Emotional or comfort eating

Many people eat when they feel any number of emotions, such as anger, anxiety, loneliness, conflict, stress, and frustration—although any emotion could, in theory, lead to what is known as displacement eating. If you are a displacement eater, you will choose to eat something instead of dealing directly with a situation.

The problem with food is that for many of us it has so many connotations with pleasure, sin, and guilt. If you do experience emotional or comfort eating, then the food you chose is unlikely to be what we might term "healthful." After all, if you are going to eat when you are lonely or stressed, would you choose to eat cauliflower or chocolate? Chickpeas or potato chips?

Boredom

Mindless eating happens often, and certainly isn't anything to do with real hunger. Research undertaken at the University of Massachusetts and published in 2006 suggested that a person's intake of food rises by as much as 71 percent when eating while watching television.

Habit

Although we might not feel hungry when it is time to eat, we often eat out of habit rather than because of genuine hunger. This approach can actually work very well, as I will explain later in section three, but eating out of habit on a regular basis isn't really an issue of hunger.

Politeness

We can often overeat simply because we feel that we should finish what is on our plates out of politeness—even if we feel full halfway through a meal.

Taste

Once again, this isn't a question of being hungry, but rather the desire to eat something from a food group that perhaps hasn't been included as part of your meal. The most obvious example is dessert: you may want to eat something sweet, even though you feel full after eating your main meal.

So you can see that while we eat for numerous reasons, real hunger is not always the primary reason. We live in plentiful times with access to a wonderful variety of food, and eating is often more of a pleasure or an emotional reaction to a situation than a response to a biochemical signal requesting fuel for the body to use as energy.

"I used to think that I didn't eat more than slim people, but I was kidding myself."

A. D.

Is being fat a modern sin?

Over the years, I have heard overweight people describe themselves —or rather, the way others treat them—in the most damning and shocking way. Their self-esteem is usually nonexistent, as living life in the fat lane can be unpleasant and demoralizing. While I have never been what might be termed "fat," I do understand what it can be like. I have been a little overweight, and I was pretty hard on myself, despite pretending that I wasn't getting bigger and hoping that no one else would notice. I carried on fooling myself until someone I worked with said no more than, "Gosh, if you don't watch out you will be a fatty!" My cover was blown, and I went on a diet that was punishing and miserable. At this point in my life I knew nothing about food and nutrition, so I drank diet cola and ate low-fat everything— and not much of it, mind you—until I lost the weight. I was hungry and tired all the time, but that fitted in nicely with my feelings of being annoyed with myself for letting myself gain weight. The diet felt like the appropriate punishment for my stupidity and gluttony. Thankfully, this all took place shortly before I enrolled on the nutrition course that led me to becoming a nutrition consultant.

Since then, I have learned how to eat, and this has saved me from a life spent either on or off a diet, counting calories, and worrying about my weight and image. I am aware of what I eat, but the way I eat is second nature to me. However, I know that if I were to take my eye off the ball, I could go back to where I was. I must stress that this does not mean that I am always on a diet, just that I have a simple template of how to eat that allows me to enjoy consistently good levels of energy as well as eating well (which means eating the kind of food that one might consider to be indulgent, too).

I have learned how to eat and this has saved me from a life spent either on or off a diet, counting calories, and worrying about my weight and image.

Some 15 years on, I have heard countless stories like my own, but usually without the happy ending. I have often wondered what it is about being overweight that is so very threatening and upsetting for people (both for those who are overweight and for those who judge them). It is my belief that being fat, overweight, chubby, wobbly, or big has come to represent something quite fundamental and causes profound discomfort in society. If being fat is a sin—and it is certainly treated as one—I think that this one sin is the manifestation of a number of others. Has being fat become synonymous with the "seven deadly sins"?

The "seven deadly sins"

Most of us have heard of the seven deadly sins, but let's look again at the list and see how being fat fits these vices. I should stress that I do not hold with these views; instead, I am interested in why our weight makes us feel so uncomfortable about ourselves.

Gluttony
Pride
Envy
Lust
Anger
Greed
Sloth

Gluttony

Being fat reveals the ultimate gluttony; some people feel that this is the physical manifestation of greed. "If you weren't greedy, then you wouldn't be fat, would you?"

Pride

This category is a little perverse, as anyone who takes pride in the way they look would surely not allow themselves to grow fat. Does being fat show a lack of pride, almost a disdain for appearances that goes against the norm?

Envy

Does someone else's weight problem make us feel superior and thus enviable? An overweight person might look at a slim person with envy, perhaps desiring their ability to eat what they like without gaining any weight.

Lust

The sin of lust suggests giving in to the "sins of the flesh," but we can also lust after food. A fat person might be judged as lustful, because they have clearly been indulging their lust for food.

Anger

I think that many fat people can be angry with themselves for letting their weight problem go on too long and allowing themselves to become fat. Other people often seem angered by their overweight peers, as they wonder how they could let themselves go to that degree.

Greed

A common assumption is that fat people eat too much — certainly more than their fair share — and their size is viewed as proof of their greed and inability to control their appetite.

Sloth

Fat people are often considered slothful, because if they were more active they simply wouldn't be fat. And since fat people can't move as fast as their slimmer, fitter counterparts, aren't they therefore slothful by comparison?

In many ways, being overweight is considered a manifestation of these sins. If being slim "and in control," which is highly prized in our society, is one end of the spectrum, being fat shows that you have needs and can't control them. When I meet people for the first time and we have a meal together, they often infer that I must have good powers of self-control, as how else would I manage not to eat the bread and stop myself from succumbing to dessert? Using that logic, overeating suggests that you have no self-control, which is considered a great failing, and instead have given in to desire.

The language of fat

As if we needed further proof that "fat is bad and thin is good," let's look at the language and words that are used to describe people who carry excess weight, some of which are more pleasant than others. This excess might be as little as a few pounds or as many as fifty or more.

Mild/innocuous

Round Voluptuous Beer belly Solid Curvy

Generous Rubenesque

Chubby Chunky Stocky

Plump

Harsh/insulting

Fatty Obese Large

Huge Roly-poly

Fatso Greedy pig

Rotund Porker Fat

Wobble-bottom Lard ass

Hefty

Heifer As big as a house

Now, let's look at the words used to describe slim people. They don't fall into mild or harsh categories (with the exception of "thin" which implies being underfed, but is still something to which overweight people might aspire):

Toned

Slim

Healthy

Thin

In proportion

Well

In shape

There aren't so many descriptive words in this list, but they are all words that are positive and pleasant and can be used in a complimentary manner, unlike the fat words, which can be (and are) used to mock and insult the overweight.

"I have heard them all and even
 the nice ones make me cringe."
H. T.

So why do we diet? It's obvious—we diet because we want to lose weight. But let's look into this in a little more depth and explore some of the reasons *why* we want to lose weight, as they are different for everyone.

I would like to think that the primary reason for anyone wanting to lose weight is concern for their long-term health. Obesity can significantly increase the incidence of several conditions, including

▸ **Type 2 diabetes**
▸ **Cardiovascular disease (heart attack and stroke)**
▸ **Some types of cancer**
▸ **Joint problems, including osteoarthritis**
▸ **Sleep apnea**
▸ **Insulin resistance**
▸ **Fatty liver disease**
▸ **Infertility and pregnancy complications**
▸ **Gallbladder disease.**

The more overweight you are, the higher your risk of developing one or more of these conditions. The risks don't kick in just when you are termed officially obese; the health issues and risks become more serious and more likely when you weigh more than the recommended weight for your height.

And while more women than men choose to diet, this does not mean that men don't need to lose weight for the same reasons, as the health complications are equally severe and present for men.

If you think that obesity applies to other people and you are just simply overweight or a little plump, does this list apply to you? Yes, it does, though not quite to the same extent.

"It won't happen to me."

Just to put things in perspective, if you smoked a pack of cigarettes every day, you might be more aware of the health risks than someone who doesn't smoke. Even if you didn't fully acknowledge the ramifications of your 20-a-day habit, you can't ignore the fact that you would be taking a big risk. Or if you drank a bottle of wine every day, again, the health issues associated with the increased level of units of alcohol might be very apparent to you, even if you largely ignored them. However, being obese can mean a 65-percent increase in the chances of experiencing chronic conditions (whereas smoking a pack of cigarettes or "heavy" drinking leads to a 25-percent increase).

It is a natural human trait to feel immortal and to think that ill health is something that happens to other people. Unless you have already experienced any of the health problems listed here, it's likely that there will be an element of "It won't happen to me" in your attitude toward your health.

Now, let's be honest here. How many people who have gained weight and then chosen to lose it again have done so primarily for health reasons?

How often do you hear people say that they want to lose weight because they are worried about fatty liver disease? Or that they want to start a diet just in case their gallbladder is adversely affected by their extra weight? I am sure that some people will recognize that the excess weight they have accumulated is potentially damaging to their health and lose weight accordingly, but the overriding motivation for most people to choose to lose weight is because of how upset they feel about being classed as fat. The long and the short of it is that most people lose weight because they feel bad about themselves, and no one is less tolerant of fat people than fat people themselves. In spite of the health risks, I remain convinced that the vast majority of people who lose weight do so because they feel self-conscious about themselves, not because they are worried about their liver or gallbladder.

Social attitudes

As we've discovered, being overweight carries with it several health risks, ranging from an increased risk of some forms of cancer to infertility and being immobile. I could list an even longer selection of health conditions, but the truth is that we don't usually look at a fat person and worry about their increased risk of cancer, or sympathize with them about how difficult it must be for them to run for a bus. Of all my consultations with clients, I can honestly say that I can count on the fingers of just one hand the number of people who have asked for advice on weight loss because they want to reduce the likelihood of a major illness. I have come to believe that our personal opinion of fat is largely governed by the fact that being fat is considered unsightly, even "wrong," in our society.

This may be an uncomfortable truth, but being fat has become far more of a cosmetic issue than a health concern.

Historically, how we look and how we present ourselves to others has been important to every civilization in the world. I think it's safe to say that our modern, media-filled world has influenced our interest in (or at least our awareness of) our looks more than ever before, and how we appear to those around us is now of enormous relevance to the majority of people to one degree or another.

Different cultures around the world have different attitudes to size, and it's easy to think that what we consider "normal" is the general attitude of our own culture. The majority of the Western world appears to favor the lean look as being an ideal to attain, while other cultures find a more rounded figure more attractive.

I remember some 18 years ago going to stay with some friends who live abroad. It was the middle of winter in Britain, and I was looking forward to sunshine and beaches. Aware that I had indulged myself over Christmas, and wanting a flat stomach for the beach, I ate carefully and didn't drink alcohol for one month prior to the trip. I duly lost weight. My friends and family at home commented on the weight loss and I remember feeling rather smug, as I had successfully lost weight while so many others seemed to struggle. It was so easy; what was all the fuss about?

My friends overseas were less impressed, however, as in their eyes I appeared thin and scrawny rather than toned and slim. Instead of compliments and support, I received pity, as my friends assumed I wasn't well. This simple example serves to illustrate how two evolved cultures hold entirely different views about size and body weight.

Why is being slim so cool?

I have already mentioned that I make no judgment about people's size, but I do witness the misery and despair that individuals who are overweight can experience when they battle with their weight.

But what's the big deal about being slim? What makes it such a cool thing to be? And how do you really feel about fat people, or about the possibility of being a fat person yourself? If being fat is a representation of the seven deadly sins, how does this translate into everyday life, and would it be too flippant to suggest that being fat is just not cool?

"I look at slim people and wonder what it must be like. They don't know what it's like to be on an eternal diet." A. D.

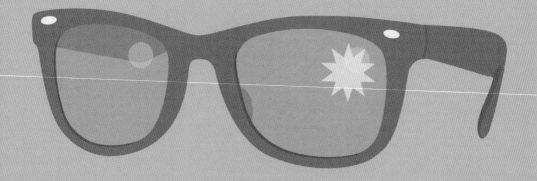

Imagine that it's a warm, sunny day after a spell of rain, and you are sitting on the patio of a country pub next to the river. It's a Sunday, and you and your boyfriend/girlfriend/husband/wife/partner are with a few close friends, having just had lunch. You are enjoying the last of your wine as you sit by the river. In the near distance is the parking lot, and you happen to glance over as a sleek car drives in. You realize that this car is something you have promised yourself that one day you will own, too. The roof is down and the body is gleaming in the sunshine; you can hear sophisticated jazz music emanating from the car as it glides into a parking space, the engine is switched off, the door opens and . . .

Now stop.

Take a few seconds and picture the type of person you might imagine would be getting out of the car. Think about how they look, what they might be wearing. So, back to the gleaming car . . .

. . . and out steps the driver, well-dressed, glossy, and . . . fat. Not "can't leave the house fat," but very, very big.

Did you imagine that? I'm sure you didn't. You see, the car is cool, but being fat isn't. In our eyes, the two don't go together. In fact, most things that are cool don't look right when they are worn, carried, or even driven by a fat person. If being slim and toned suggests that you are cool, then the opposite is true for being fat. The presenting impression many people have when they see a fat person is just that: they are fat. Imagine how that perspective might make people worry about getting fat, or even gaining weight. Fat is so uncool and feared that people who are not fat may go to seemingly extreme measures to avoid it.

"I promised myself that I would buy a chic navy suit for my daughter's graduation. But what's the point when you are my size?" M. C.

"I look at the clothing catalogs for the larger figure and even I am appalled by how the clothes look." **H. T.**

Each of us has a highly personal opinion of what it means to be fat, and I wonder to what extent it influences the way that we eat, even if we don't need to lose weight. I have heard from thousands of clients over the years who have dieted at a time when they didn't need to, and it is my belief that the desire to be slim distorts the way we look at ourselves. This mild body dysmorphia, or imagined body defect, is obviously unhealthy, and if we diet when it's not necessary simply because our mind tells us that we need to be slimmer, then this interferes with our natural metabolic rate (pp.40–43) and begins a cycle of losing and gaining weight that can last a lifetime.

So could it be that it's not the food we eat or the diets that are making us fat; it's actually the process of dieting itself?

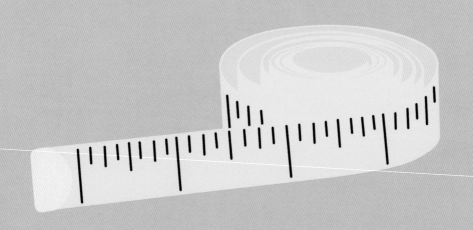

Genetics, and accepting our fate Genetics plays an important role in all aspects of our physical makeup. Although we are all probably quite familiar with the facial resemblances and character traits that we share with our parents, siblings, and offspring, to what extent might our parents' weight influence our own size?

The link between genetics and weight is the subject of ongoing research, and I daresay that in the future scientists will be able to adapt our genes so that we can all be slim, gifted, and intelligent. But for now, what are we stuck with? Our individual genetic makeup can affect our overall weight by anywhere between 40 and 70 percent, so if you have parents who are overweight, you may well have to do the best you can with the hand that you have been dealt.

Genetics doesn't just affect how heavy we are, it also influences the areas where fat can accumulate on our bodies. So if your mother tends to gain weight around her hips, the chances are that you may, too. Or if your father is an apple shape, the chances are higher that you might be, too—but only if you gain weight.

Is it too late to change your fate?

I do wonder about the extent to which we either simply accept our genetic fate, or try to battle against what is largely predestined. There has to be a balance between the two extremes of doing nothing to prevent weight gain and trying everything to avoid it.

If genetics predetermines as much as 70 percent of your weight, and your parents are overweight, then in theory it would seem futile for you to keep trying to lose the weight. But think again. Just how much of what your parents weigh is attributable to their genes, and how much is due to their own issues with eating?

I believe that while diets work, dieting doesn't, and the whole process of dieting in the way that we often do (that is, to get results, fast) actually upsets our metabolic rate. You've read in section one about the way in which our metabolism responds to a reduction in calorie intake (pp.40–42); and, as I have mentioned, many people with current weight problems started dieting when they were young, perhaps in their teens or 20s. It follows that many people will have dieted when they didn't need to, perhaps to try to reach some unattainable goal or conform to social pressure, which itself can lead to problems in the longer term.

So how can you tell if the weight your parents are carrying around is due to their own genetics or to poor eating habits? Obviously it's not going to be easy to pinpoint which additional pound you put on is due to your ancestors or to overindulging at Christmas, so you will have to trust your own judgment on this one.

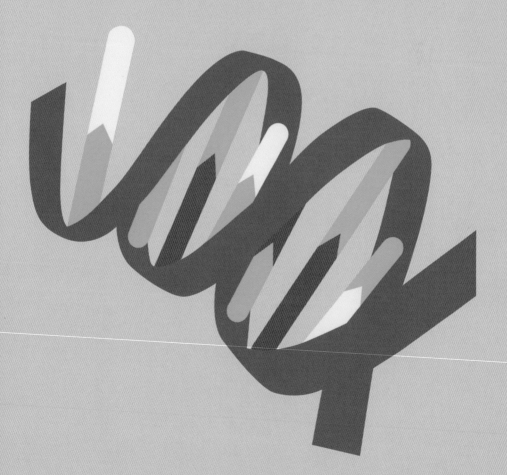

Media advertising and the food industry

Information about food is communicated in many ways, but most of what we know about food comes from advertisements and is therefore commercially driven. The power of advertising is extraordinary, as what we see portrayed in those slick, clever 30-second television commercials or slick magazine or billboard ads can often enter the national psyche.

For example, if I ask you to name a low-fat yogurt, there is a high probability that you will be able to name a best-selling product, even if you have never eaten or bought one before. The same goes for canned sweetcorn or low-fat breakfast cereal; I am sure you can quickly recall a brand and the individual product, whether you love or hate sweetcorn or low-fat cereal. Even the music that is used in television advertising can remind us of a particular product. The average person—if asked to hum a tune from *Lakmé*, a seldom-performed opera by Léo Delibes—would probably draw a blank. Yet a few years ago, the 'Flower Duet' from that opera was used in a TV commercial for a leading British airline and worked its way into the public consciousness—its beguiling strains conjuring up the pleasure of taking to the skies. We shouldn't underestimate the power of advertising in influencing what we buy, and of course, what we choose to eat.

Creating a problem to solve

One of the most effective ways in which the food industry markets a product is to present it as a solution to a problem. Although the problem is unlikely to exist in the first place, the marketing suggests it does so that we can buy into the solution by purchasing the product. In the food business, it is largely accepted that consumers decide which foods to buy for three reasons: taste, value, and health. You might buy a food for any combination of these reasons; and, putting price aside, health and taste have always been at odds with one another. Or that's what the food industry would have us believe. Fruit is healthful, as are vegetables, and they taste good (well, not all of them, but most of them). However, there isn't much markup on fresh produce, so food marketing concentrates on foods that have been processed in some way, which adds commercial value and allows for a hefty profit margin (which, in turn, funds the advertising). Corn, for example, is healthful, low in fat, and rich in nutrients, but in its simplest form it is perhaps not the first thing you might think of to eat for breakfast. If the corn is picked, processed, and packaged, however, it becomes a high-value and appealing breakfast cereal that has the advantage of being quick and easy to consume.

Having breakfast never used to be a problem. Our great-grandparents were unaware that the time it took them to prepare and eat their breakfast could actually be a problem. So to encourage society to change its eating habits, the food industry suggested that breakfast was a time-consuming, complicated meal and offered up cereal as the solution—usually without having to say that breakfast was a problem in the first place. Soon this notion was generally accepted and, in time, became part of the everyone's psyche.

"I am a sucker for advertisements. If there's a chance it might work to make me thin, I'll try it. What have I got to lose?"

M. L.

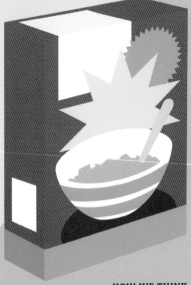

Manipulating the consumer's choice

If we apply this approach to low-fat food, most advertisers promise that you can eat their product without feeling guilty, or that you can eat it often, as it's low in fat. This low-fat claim is often promoted because we are generally aware that eating too many full-fat foods isn't a healthy option, as they can be "fattening." Our obsession with weight is a gift to the food industry, because it can sell foods that have the aura of being healthful by virtue of the fact that they are low in fat. So the subliminal message of low-fat food is that it is good for us (especially if it is a low-fat version of something that would otherwise contain fat, or perhaps isn't part of what we might consider to be "a diet food"). The advertising never directly states that low-fat food is good for us; instead, it relies on our misapprehension that full fat is always bad for us. Having read about blood glucose in section one, you will know that low-fat foods can create glucose rapidly (p.20), which leads to an increase in insulin levels and therefore easily contributes to fat stores in the body. This doesn't mean that low-fat or full-fat foods are better or worse for us—that's a different issue, which we will tackle in section three—but if you are watching your weight, then a vague notion that eating full-fat food is going to make you fat will inevitably make you choose the low-fat version.

Think about it: no advertisement for low-fat food actually says that you can eat it without becoming fat, does it? Advertisers rely on what is generally accepted—that eating some foods makes you fat—and then imply that you can eat their food and not gain weight.

Right?
Wrong.

Research suggests that if we believe a food to be nonfattening, "good," or even "allowed," we eat far more of it, in the belief that it doesn't count against us. If we think, for example, that eating a full-fat dessert is a sin and something that is fundamentally wrong, we also assume that we can eat more of a low-fat, artificially sweetened version of that dessert in a guilt-free way. However, eating the low-fat dessert inevitably perpetuates your desire for sweet foods, which means that at some point you relent and opt for the real thing, and you gain weight. Once you gain weight, you resort to the artificial version, and soon your desire for the full-fat version surfaces again …

This desire, or craving, as the food industry would prefer us to think of it, is something that we have been conditioned into thinking is wrong, a desire that has to be beaten. And you can beat it by eating the version that the industry promotes instead.

To push the point a little further, is getting into your car to drive home after having drunk a bottle of wine a mistake? Of course it is. But what if you have drunk only half a bottle? Is it less of a mistake than having a whole bottle? Well, yes, but is it right? Of course it isn't. Yet one can justify it, if one is so minded, along the lines of "Surely it's better than driving after having had a whole bottle?" If you have ever wondered, "Surely low fat is better than full fat?"—and the chances are that you have—to what extent might you have been justifying your food choice by comparing it to its wicked alternative? (We will look more closely at the issue of "Surely it's better than …?" in section three.)

You may wish to reflect on your beliefs about food and whether they will serve you well in the future. Think about where those beliefs come from; and, given what you now know about how the body works, perhaps you might see how the foods that you eat have contributed, or will contribute, to potential weight issues in the future.

I maintain that it is this sort of confusion that perpetuates the misconception that many foods are essentially bad for us, that eating is a problem, and that we are gluttons who are out of control. My experience tells me that this belief contributes to our weight issues, because we make what are essentially poor food choices.

I hope that you can now see that it is the misguided attitudes we glean from product advertising, and not the foods themselves, that contribute to a large degree of ignorance about our relationship with food.

Other subliminal influences As we have seen,

product advertising and the media greatly influence our ideas about food. In Britain and some other countries, food advertising aimed at children is subject to strict regulations regarding both the content and when the ads can be broadcast, which highlights what a powerful influence advertising has on young minds.

But now that we are all grown up, what other factors influence our thoughts about food, and just how independently minded are we when it comes to eating?

Families

From an early age, we are conditioned to eat in the same way that our family does. If your family happens to think that eating very large portions is normal, then you might, too. Or if your mother cooks food in a certain way, then for you, that's the way it's done and that's how you are likely to cook it, too. I remember being invited to Thanksgiving with newly married American friends. This was the first time the bride had cooked for her own, and now extended, family. When the turkey was ready, she presented it at the table to puzzled looks: she had cut the bird straight down the middle and placed the two symmetrical halves on the serving platter. When her extended family asked her why she had done that, she replied, "But this is the way it's done. After all, Mom has always done it this way." When her mother stopped laughing, she explained to everyone that her own oven was so small that the only way she could cook a large turkey was to cut it in half and roast it in separate trays. Apart from being a rather amusing anecdote, it demonstrates how we accept much of what happens in our own homes as being normal, and do so often without question.

I think it's common for us to give more weight to comments made by our parents and siblings than we would to strangers' comments. I am sure that I am not alone in being sensitive about what my family says to me. If your parents or a sibling, for example, suggests that you need to lose weight, you are more likely to listen and react (in one way or the other). I remember how one client, who had lost and gained weight throughout her adult life, eventually pinpointed the start of this unhappy cycle to witnessing the teasing that her elder sister received when she gained weight in her late teens. Although my client wasn't overweight herself, she started to diet, albeit gently at first. But as her sibling gained weight, she became increasingly anxious about being teased and adopted a restrictive diet and strenuous exercise routine. On the surface one could argue (and indeed, my client did) that eating well and exercising were all in the name of good health, but that wasn't her true motivating factor. My client's actions forced her metabolism to sense impending famine, and it reacted as it is programmed to do (pp.40–43). She began a lifetime of weight problems, both physiological and psychological.

"The fact that I am overweight is the 'elephant in the room' with my mother. She spent my childhood telling me not to eat in case I got fat. Now that I am, she says nothing." **A. C.**

Many of the views your family hold will be generational, and we must understand that however our ancestors ate 20 or even 100 years ago, life and food are different now. Whatever eating plan you follow has to be practical, affordable, and realistic. This is not to say that our parents or grandparents got it wrong, but they will be the first to tell you how different things are today than when they were younger.

Friends, colleagues, and pack mentality

We shouldn't think that we are affected only by our family's habits and opinions, as any group that we are part of will have a degree of influence on our behavior if we let it. Basic animal psychology highlights "pack mentality," and human beings can develop this way of thinking as easily as other animals. When it comes to dieting, research suggests that people who diet as part of a group lose more weight than those who go it alone. The pack mentality may well inject a note of competitive dieting as people try to outdo one another, but also I suspect that individuals dare not be the only one in the group to fail or the one to lose the least amount of weight. I should add that the person who loses the most weight in a group of dieters often has the most to lose to begin with, and there is a good chance that their metabolic rate will suffer as a result. So losing more weight than others isn't quite the glowing achievement it might seem.

By the same token, eating in a group often means that you eat more than you normally would. If you regularly eat lunch with a group of work colleagues, it's likely that any of the comments given here that they might make will influence your food choices.

> You deserve it. It's been a long week.

> Go on: I will if you will.

> Let's have dessert. I'm in no rush to get back to the office.

Of course, there is nothing wrong with any of these statements, but all too often peer encouragement, never mind peer pressure, can persuade us to change the way we eat simply so that we fit in. We are all susceptible to the moods and attitudes of the people around us. And when it comes to diet and food, everyone around you is an expert, especially about what you eat, or should be eating.

I often tell clients who are following a new food plan not to tell anyone else, simply because they will get comments that may or may not be encouraging. Casual asides such as "I tried that; it didn't work" or "I am sure I read that this food is bad for you" can sow seeds of doubt that can sabotage anyone who isn't resolute in their intentions.

Aside from work colleagues, there are other groups of people that we all find ourselves part of. Friends are perhaps the most obvious influence; and, like work colleagues and family, they also watch television and look at magazines, newspapers, and websites. Their knowledge about food is therefore as much affected by popular culture as anyone else's, but in a group, people inevitably talk and share ideas, and it's easy to take on board the comments and attitudes of that group. If you have a group of friends who meet in a bar once a week and tend to drink a little more than you would ideally like, it is hard to cut down on drinking without highlighting your reduced intake and drawing attention to the amount that everyone else generally drinks. In addition, some friends are more persuasive than others when you don't really want to drink or eat something. Research shows that when people eat with friends, they eat as much as 35 percent more food than when they eat alone or with strangers.

I am not suggesting that you abandon your social life or always eat alone, but being aware of how other people's eating habits can influence yours can only be a good thing. Understanding this will certainly help you in realizing your own values and what really matters to you when it comes to food.

Eating out and dieting

Many clients who come to me for advice about how to eat often claim that they can't follow a particular food plan because they usually eat out, for either work or social reasons. They believe that because they eat out so often they aren't in control of what they eat, and thus can't "diet." As I don't subscribe to the old-fashioned traditional method of dieting, I work to show clients how to adopt a way of eating that can be used at all times and in all situations, including eating out.

There is a misconception that eating out is the death of a good food plan, and if that's what you believe, it becomes true every time you eat out. If eating out is a rare treat, I suggest you enjoy the evening and eat food that you wouldn't normally eat at home (although this doesn't necessarily mean that you have to eat your own body weight just because you aren't at home).

Eating (or drinking) is, of course, to be enjoyed and shared with friends and family, and used to grease social wheels. This is not to say that enjoyment can't come from the company you share as well as the food you eat, but this is, of course, more easily said than done. There is still a way to be part of a group without taking on everything that other people think about food, but we will look into this in more detail in section three.

Have we got too many choices?

I have often heard it said, "The more the alternatives, the more difficult the choice." And what a choice it is when it comes to what we eat. As the expression goes, we are "spoiled for choice."

Consumerism features heavily in the Western world, and perhaps the primary attribute of a consumer-led economy is choice. Giving customers a choice is paramount for manufacturers, distributors, and retailers, and having a wide choice of goods available is considered an achievement. I am sure that the thinking behind this includes the concept that having such a variety of goods to choose from empowers the consumer, but does it really? And are the choices that we have to make—not just in the supermarket, but everywhere in the food world—simply muddying the waters? Psychologists refer to the plethora of choices we have as "consumer vertigo," because it often leads to confusion. I also believe that it can contribute to a level of unhappiness and dissatisfaction, as we invariably wonder what else we could and should be doing, buying, and even eating.

Psychologists refer to the plethora of choices we have as "consumer vertigo," because it often leads to confusion.

Consumer vertigo

If you have ever been on a diet, you will be familiar with the concept of cravings and longings. Imagine that you have been on a calorie-controlled diet for a couple of weeks; it's dull and uneventful, yet you are losing weight. At this point, it's amazing how the choice of foods available to you can take on an extraordinary status. As you have been dieting, you might think you deserve a treat, but you dare not risk eating an indulgent cookie coated with chocolate and filled with pieces of caramel, as your diet would be ruined after all your hard work and denial. Yet the allure of the cookie grows and takes on unnatural proportions in your mind. If you finally give in and eat the cookie, does it actually deliver what it promised? Is it worth it?

That looks good. Double chocolate; I wonder how many calories …?

Oh, it's got caramel in it as well. I love caramel. Maybe I could have just one, it's only 340 calories and I could skip dinner …

It looks so good, and eating it would be so nice: all that chocolate melting …

… and it's got oats in it, oats are good for you, I read that somewhere ….

That was so good, I feel better now. Hmmm. But all those calories …

Why did I do that?

That's just typical of me. It didn't even taste that good!

I can't believe I ate that cookie; it was such a stupid thing to do. After all my hard work, I had to go and ruin it …

Needless to say, eating the chocolate-caramel cookie (Or cookies—after all, why stop at one? You have ruined it now so you might as well carry on and eat more) might make you feel any number of emotions in the moment, including rebelliousness, indulgence, and a sense of having deserved it. But a couple of hours later, how does eating the cookie make you feel? Does your decision to go with that choice still feel quite so worthwhile?

The dissatisfaction of choice

The reality is that some of the food choices we make simply don't match up to their tempting promises. We do know this, yet we allow ourselves to be caught up in very short-term emotions at the expense of long-term gains.

It's worth bearing in mind that the average supermarket stocks 30,000 or more different items, and in each category several—sometimes dozens—of similar products are offered. Moreover, many thousand new products are launched each year; and in order to have any chance of success, a new product has to be supported and promoted, not only in the store itself but also in the wider world. This means that the new product has to be marketed or discounted (perhaps by way of a special offer) so that it grabs our attention. We have already looked at the issue of advertising and marketing (pp.74–77), and you will know that perhaps the most effective way to sell products is to draw them into the national psyche by one means or another.

If we use the analogy of a bank account again to express this dichotomy, dieting is the equivalent of managing your finances to reduce an overdraft little by little, only to blow the good intentions and spend what you have saved on a piece of clothing. I am sure that we have all done this, or something like it, at some point and probably justified the purchase: "It was on sale, and I could do with some shirts. I can always wear them." But let's be completely honest: How much of what you have bought in the past, all justified in the usual way,

has been worthwhile? If you look at your wardrobe, or CD or DVD collection, I can guarantee that a good proportion of it will have been a waste—poor purchases that haven't lived up to their initial promises. However, you can still wear a shirt or watch a DVD, even if it wasn't worth it, but when it comes to food, the choice of the cookie is forgotten, the pleasure was momentary, yet the results affected the way you behaved and even the way you ate for some time afterward.

Consumer vertigo can color our judgment so that the very idea of having choices can distract us from what we have carefully planned.

Portion control: How much is too much?

I have a very dear friend whose figure is undeniably on the larger side. While we were on vacation together one year, she happened to comment after lunch one day that the reason I was slim was because I didn't eat much. At that precise moment I was thinking that the reason she was overweight was because she ate so much. We had both eaten the same lunch with the same dishes, yet I hadn't finished all of my meal and she had cleared her plate. She hadn't exercised that morning, so she was no hungrier than usual. It was simply that her idea of a normal portion size differed from my own. This story serves to illustrate that portion size is entirely personal, and that your idea of a normal portion size may differ quite markedly from that of someone else.

Our appetite obviously plays a role in this issue; but, putting that aside, how is it that we have such differing opinions about portion control? I am sure that there are several explanations, but my feeling is that the might of the food industry in general, and the commercialization of foods in particular, are major factors.

I have touched already on three primary reasons that drive consumers to choose food: taste, health benefits, and price. It's the last that I feel is a major influence on portion size, as larger amounts of food for sale at a given price may offer better value. This may seem obvious, but what is less apparent is that images of large quantities of food can start to filter into our minds, which inevitably influences the amount of food that we consider to be normal. In other words, the more we get for our money is considered to be good value, and this has warped our sense of a normal portion size.

The super-size trend

This increase in portion size was probably first seen on a mass scale in the United States in 1993, when McDonald's introduced "dino size" portions to tie with the launch of the movie *Jurassic Park*. After the promotion, this portion size was retained, but was known as "super size" until it was phased out in 2004. A study published in 2002 in the *American Journal of Public Health* also found that "bakers are using larger muffin tins" and that "fast-food restaurants are using larger French fry and drink containers." It was even found that the cup holders built into new cars were larger than a decade earlier. Visually, this has to have an impact on how we now see smaller portions, as they can look puny— even poor value—and medium-size portions suddenly seem less bulky. Could it be that the advent of super-size portions makes the large option, which used to be the biggest offered, look somewhat like the disciplined choice? Even if you don't choose the super-size portions, have your expectations increased accordingly, so that you now eat more anyway?

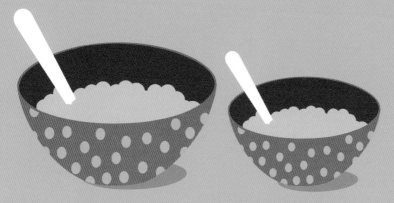

The drive to offer good value affects food advertising also. Restaurant chains and processed food products often carry images of plates covered with generous servings of food to suggest good value. Take a moment and think about what you believe a "normal" main-course portion size should look like. I am confident that if you were to look at images of portions from 30 years ago, you might consider them to be small, even if you feel that today's offerings are too large.

Needless to say, this is bound to change how much we eat, and I believe that we eat more than we need to. The way to keep an eye on this tendency to overeat is to be more savvy about how much food we put on our plate, which we will cover in detail in section three.

Diet and gender

Weight-loss solutions have been around now for a few hundred years in one form or another, but they perhaps first became popular and entered the mainstream in the late nineteenth century after a British undertaker, William Banting, advocated a new diet plan. Banting, who had become so grossly overweight that he was unable even to bend down to tie his shoelaces, was advised by his doctor to continue to eat protein and fat and reduce his intake of carbohydrates. Having lost substantial amounts of weight by adhering to the plan, Banting then published his *Letter on Corpulence* in 1862. People all over Britain followed Banting's written advice, which would now be termed a "fad diet." His diet proved so popular that it was often referred to as "the Banting diet."

Women and dieting

We don't know what proportion of Banting's followers were female, but I think that it is a fair assumption that more than half of them would have been women. Certainly, the majority of people who are on a diet of some form or another today are women, a fact underlined by the attention paid to women's weight and shape in our popular press. Female celebrities are mocked for their weight gain, cheered for their weight loss, and then pitied if they gain it again. Headlines such as those opposite are commonplace now. Statistics vary enormously, but they suggest that, at any one time, as much as 65 percent of the adult population in Britain is on a diet of one type or another, irrespective of whether that man or woman needs to lose weight or not. Young women aged between 18 and 24 fare the same, and the statistics also suggest that 40 percent of girls who are younger than 18 have already tried a diet, or feel that they ought to go on a diet.

The pressure on women to be slim is enormous, and as it now seems to be an obsession in the popular press it would be hard for any woman to remain unaffected by this pressure. Over the years, I have asked many clients why they wanted to lose weight. Many young women felt that they wouldn't find a boyfriend if they were overweight, while others felt that success in any professional field would elude them unless they were slim. The expectations of society are not easy to ignore.

CELEBRITY IN CELLULITE SHOCK

Is she putting it all back on?

Fears grow for lead singer's health as she becomes too thin

Men and dieting

When I first started to practice as a nutrition consultant, my clients were almost exclusively female. The occasional man would be dragged along by the woman in his life to see me, but few, if any, men came of their own accord. Even though weight loss is just one area that I am consulted about, one could be forgiven for thinking that men had no conditions resulting from their general diet that might benefit from an expert nutritional analysis.

In the space of just ten years this situation has changed, and now it is not unusual for men to visit the clinic for dietary advice. When I give talks or hold workshops, there are often men in the audience, and they, too, are becoming increasingly interested in their diet.

This is, of course, a good thing, as my experience suggests that many men don't make any changes to their diet unless they have suffered some sort of health problem or illness. The reality is that men don't live with the same amount of social pressure that women live with when it comes to size and shape.

However, there is an increasing amount of pressure on men to conform to a physical ideal, and images of well-toned, slim men that were once found only on the front of health magazines are now becoming increasingly common in the popular press as well. My main interest in men and dieting is that it is seems inevitable that, in time, increasing numbers of men will fall into the same diet trap as women if they chase a physical ideal.

> "I never used to think about weight until my girlfriend started asking why I didn't have abs."
> M. K.

I have worked with many men over the years who have needed to lose weight; and, somewhat frustratingly for women, they all seem to do so with ease and excellent results the first time around. This has nothing to do with some strange gender-specific genetic ability, but is simply because those men have never been on a diet before. Their metabolic rates have not been affected by repeated cycles of feast and famine; and, equally importantly, they have not been frustrated by the success and subsequent failure of previous diets. As diets and the dream of perfected bodies have not previously been on their radar, men are usually happy to take on the advice and apply it without question. As a result, they can be a little smug when the weight comes off. "What s the big fuss about? I did it easily." Yet they are less smug when the weight goes back on and they have to start another diet again.

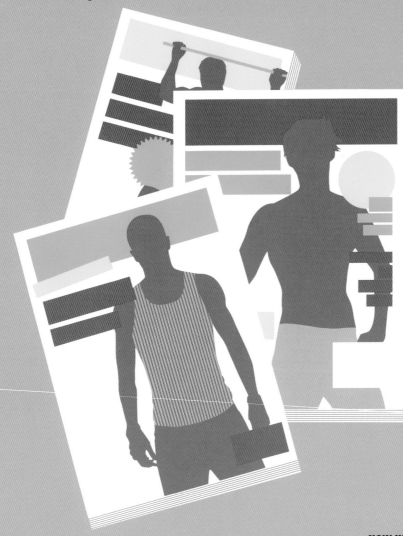

Why diets work but dieting doesn't

All diets work—in isolation, that is. Whether you are eating only soup, avoiding wheat or some other food that a specialist lab—having examined your blood under a microscope—says you are allergic to, eating only protein or perhaps raw food grown by vegan farmers, so long as you buy into the "science" or story behind the diet and follow the instructions, you will inevitably lose weight in the short term. Many people thrive on a given plan to follow, possibly because it imposes limits or a set of rules that remove any doubt or room for mistakes, which can be pleasing.

For anyone who is reading this book and doesn't need to lose weight, you may well wonder why someone wouldn't stick to a plan if it really is that successful. So let me explain what happens to the average dieter who follows what they consider to be an "easy" diet.

Having tried to lose weight and done so successfully on more than one occasion, the average dieter finds that the weight creeps back on. Perhaps there were mitigating circumstances, such as a stressful period of time (comfort eating), or an illness that meant the dieter was at home for a period of time (comfort eating and inactivity), but whatever the reasons, the dieter is back to wanting, or needing, to lose weight. Having seen an extract of a book in a national newspaper claiming that a particular diet is the secret of Hollywood celebrities, the dieter buys that diet book and reads it, and it all makes sense and seems so easy. So the dieter undertakes the plan and it works. The dieter starts to feel all the things that one benefits from when one loses weight: better sleep, more energy, and more attention and compliments from others. The dieter's self-esteem increases . . . When the desired weight is reached, it is inevitable that real life will kick in. Perhaps, having avoided wheat, eaten only protein, or not eaten different food groups at the same meal, the dieter finds him- or herself in a situation in which only wheat and dairy or carbohydrates are available. Having lost the weight, the dieter may wonder if it could hurt to have just a little of these "forbidden" foods, and so he or she does . . . Now, having broken the diet once, the dieter will do so again—not every day, of course, just every now and again, perhaps. The reasons for having been so desperate to lose weight in the first place are no longer quite so apparent, and the dieter can't quite remember how he or she felt previously because the discomfort and shame of being overweight has dimmed. So a little weight comes back on, although the dieter is determined to go back on the plan sometime soon. Anyway, a few pounds may have crept back on, but no one has said anything, so the dieter seems to have gotten away with it. And little by little, even more weight comes back on . . .

Many dieters view "easy" diets as a quick way out: if they put the weight back on, the diet is their get-out-of-jail-free card. Because it is so easy, they go back to their old eating habits and simply return to a diet plan whenever it suits them. In this way the dieter stays stuck in a rut of—easy or otherwise—diet and eat, boom or bust.

The attraction of fad diets

Many years ago, one of the very first books I read about food and nutrition advocated eating separate food groups at different times. For some reason, this way of eating is called "food combining," which is odd, as it is actually more like "food separating." Anyway, I read the book and I was completely convinced that the foods I was eating were "fighting" in my stomach. All I had to do was to eat carbohydrates separately from protein, and wait three hours after eating any fruit before eating protein, or vice versa.

Even though I didn't need to lose weight and had adopted this way of eating in an effort to be healthy, I did lose weight. In retrospect, I understand that this was simply because I bought into a set of rules to follow, which included a period of time during which I felt that I wasn't allowed to eat (the three hours between protein and fruit).

In other words, the rules that I followed encouraged me to eat less, and I was completely sold on the whole thing. I now feel that there is no real science behind food combining, although this is not the place to go into that issue in depth. For one reason or another, I ate less and I lost weight. I was also hungry for much of the day, and I checked my watch constantly, hoping that the three hours had passed and I could eat some protein (or was it fruit?). Either way, I was hungry and I lost weight. It was the first time that I had experienced the pleasure that weight loss brought with it, and the admiring looks and comments about how "good" I was being.

The process of imposing rules as part of a diet works to get us to eat less. The more compelling the story, the more likely we are to buy into it.

This is a perfect example of how the process of imposing rules as part of a diet works to get us to eat less. The more compelling the story, the more likely we are to buy into it.

Throughout my years in practice, I have been asked to comment on diets that claim to be based on the geographical origins of your ancestors, your blood type, metabolic type, or temperament. I am sure that had I read every diet book, complete with case histories and tales of weight loss linked to some aspect of biochemistry, I would be convinced enough to embark on that food plan. It's even better if the reason why the plan works can be linked to something that has previously been overlooked; perhaps the writer discovered it by accident or, even better, someone tried to stop him or her from revealing this secret to the world. The more obscure the diet, the more likely we are to feel that we have stumbled upon something fresh that will help us to lose weight forever. If it's all about eating protein and that's what you concentrate on from now on, good for you. Or if it's a plan based on your geographical ancestry and you should avoid dairy or wheat, and you do, that's fine—as long as it works. But, you and I both know that this scenario is neither realistic nor practical.

The lure of the detox plan

I have learned to be suspicious of detox plans, and every January, when some new plan comes along that claims to detox the body, I often feel bewildered. The truth is that you and I are detoxifying right now. As you read this, your liver is diligently breaking down the toxins that you have ingested from food, drink, and the environment, and you can help your liver by eating plenty of fresh fruits and vegetables and by making sure that you aren't dehydrated. These two simple things are almost as much as you can do to benefit the liver; what you don't need to do is to starve yourself by existing on juice or soup alone in order that your liver and system can "have a rest."

The detox movement plays right into the misleading notion that your usual food choices are toxic and wrong and a detox will show you the road to cleanliness. I am sure that you can see the religious inference here, which is highlighted by the suffering that these detox plans entail. The idea of detoxing to become "clean" again is compelling, to say the least, and meets many needs, not least the guilt that we feel after indulging in food, which can be linked back to the seven deadly sins (pp.62–63). In this case, the detox diet is the nutritional equivalent of sackcloth and a confessional all rolled into a week- or month-long plan that can't realistically be sustained for any longer. Inevitably you will go back to your normal eating pattern, and the weight that has been lost will creep back. The detox plan, although often rigorous, is nothing more than a diet masquerading as a way to detoxify your system.

The detox movement plays right into the misleading notion that your usual food choices are toxic and wrong and a detox will show you the road to cleanliness.

Interestingly enough, it's in January that detox plans are most popular. They offer a one-stop solution to the problems brought about by having overeaten the previous month. Just for a moment, I want you to imagine that there is no such thing as a detox diet, no rigorous plan to help you purge after the December excess. I maintain that it is the existence of the detox diet that encourages some people to overeat in the first place.

> ## "There isn't a diet I haven't tried. You name it, I have done it."
> ### K. H.

If we use the money analogy again, a detox plan is like indulgent parents who can afford to bail out their overspending child despite extracting a promise from the son or daughter that this is absolutely, definitely, the very last time that they will waste so much money. The parents may be angry and admonish the child, but they do make things better, at least for now. The question has to be asked, though: If it were not for the wealthy and indulgent parents, would the child have overspent in the first place? Yes, possibly once, but after that? I suspect it would be far more unlikely.

Or to put it another way, looking at recent economic events, the worldwide financial crisis has been blamed on the "credit crunch." The notion that our economies rely upon credit has now forced many people to be mindful about the way they spend, as they may not be able to borrow money to make larger purchases that seemed, until relatively recently, quite normal. The detox diet is like credit: we think we can borrow against our future by overeating now. Yet we now know from reading in section one about how our metabolic rate works that our bodies don't operate this way.

High-protein diets

Another problem with strict diets is that certain foods can take on a new significance and attraction, which they wouldn't do normally. Phrases such as "Am I allowed this?" start entering a dieter's vocabulary. An example of this is protein-only diets. The dieter on a high-protein diet can eat bacon and eggs for breakfast and carry on eating protein all day long, as long as he or she avoids bread and potatoes and steers clear of fruit, which is discouraged. The dieter is astonished at how quickly the weight disappears, yet just two weeks into this diet and, having resisted the temptation of a piece of toast or a bowl of fresh berries, he or she finds that the desire for these foods grows and grows. Inevitably, at some point, the high-protein dieter will succumb and eat the toast or the berries, feel like he or she has blown the diet, carry on eating "disallowed" foods until the weight comes back, and start all over again. This cycle is all because the toast or the berries weren't allowed to begin with.

Another problem with strict diets is that certain foods can take on a new significance and attraction, which they wouldn't do normally.

The calorie conundrum

Diets that focus on calories have the same disadvantages as high-protein plans: Some foods aren't allowed, or at least we don't allow ourselves to have them because why would we waste so many of our calorie allowance on nuts, for instance?

The calorie scoring that calorie-controlled diets favor has led to the misconception that some foods are "fattening" and some are not. Calories count, of course they do, but they also introduce a number to everything we eat or drink that bears no relation to the beneficial value of a food , so they can create a potentially false view of what we should eat. We are told that the average adult male requires 2,550 calories per day and the average female needs 1,940 calories. On average, to lose one pound of fat a week, we would have to eat around 500 fewer calories every day.

When I was studying nutrition, one of my lecturers espoused the benefit of eating nuts, and several people in the lecture hall asked, "But aren't they fattening?" Let's take a moment to examine this issue, as I think it will help us to understand the underlying problem with the issue of counting calories. A dieter who has gained weight decides to follow a traditional calorie-controlled diet. Now that an upper limit of calories has been set, the dieter sticks to a reduced number of calories and loses some weight. It's worth bearing in mind that fat contains approximately nine calories per gram, and carbohydrates contain around four calories per gram. After a while, the dieter will work out that, rather than use up some of the daily calorie allowance on fat, he or she can eat lots of carbohydrates instead. After all, why eat a palmful of walnuts and consume 200 calories when you can spend the same 200 calories on, say, a butterscotch pudding? The pudding is ready-made and comes from a low-fat, and thus lower-calorie, food range that is promoted and marketed to encourage you to have the foods you want, and assumes that you like the idea of a processed, sugar-laden pudding.

If we look at the nutritional value of each offering, there is little competition. The walnuts are a source of (omega 3) essential fats, which help to boost your metabolic rate and contain an array of nutrients and protein, which converts from food to glucose slowly. The pudding offers some nutrients, sugar, and artificial sweeteners; it contains negligible fat and protein, but plenty of carbohydrates. All this information is irrelevant to the dieter, since the pudding looks indulgent and the sort of thing that wouldn't normally be allowed on a diet. Furthermore, the pudding looks more substantial than the walnuts, so it appears as if there is more food available for the same calories. This way of thinking is almost impossible to avoid when you are guided by calories alone.

The cost of counting calories

So the premise of calorie-controlled diets is that we are supposed to have huge appetites and a capacity to eat too much, but we can keep gorging as long as we eat only low-fat and thus lower-calorie foods. Such diets do nothing to reduce our natural appetite, for food invariably creates glucose quite rapidly, leading to a subsequent low that we experience as hunger.

Because breakfast is the first meal of the day, what we eat can set the scene for how we eat for the rest of the day. So let's compare a breakfast containing few calories with one that has far more.

A typical low-fat (and lower-calorie) breakfast of cereal with skim milk and a cup of black coffee is a classic way of starting off the day using as few calories as possible. (You would be "allowed" bacon and eggs for breakfast on a calorie-controlled diet, but that's something that no calorie-counter would do, as it would use up a large proportion of your allowance too early in the day.) The cereal, however, is processed and therefore a simple carbohydrate, and since it is also low in fat and protein it is converted from food into glucose quite rapidly by the digestive process. You will know from reading section one that when levels of glucose in the blood rise, the pancreas responds by secreting insulin to encourage glucose into the cells or sweep it away into storage, ensuring that glucose levels stay below the level at which they may cause damage to the cells. The caffeine from your cup of coffee also contributes to an increase in glucose levels in the short term (p.37), but as the excess is swept away your energy levels drop and you feel hungry again. But, because you are following a diet, you expect to be hungry, and you regard it as a reminder that you are on a weight-loss plan. Your thoughts turn to what you can eat without using up too many calories, and away you go again.

So however miraculous the diet was to begin with, and whatever it was based on, these factors are ultimately irrelevant if the diet requires you to eat particular foods in a way that is too far removed from what or how you normally eat. This flaw is not apparent in any individual diets, nor is it a flaw in us that has to be conquered; the flaw is in dieting itself. The whole process of dieting is completely opposed to the way the body works, and until we fully understand and accept that, we are still caught in the diet trap.

Confused dieting

The fervor that many people experience when they follow a diet can border on being religious in its intensity, as their diet delivers hope, advice, and a welcome structure to eating. I have found that any diet or eating plan that is fronted by a media-friendly celebrity or public figure is well documented. As a result of the publicity, everyone seems to think that the celebrity is an expert on dieting. We have had new diet plans from some rather unexpected sources over the past 20 years, including a former British Chancellor of the Exchequer, a high-profile literary agent, a gourmand film producer, and a brainy game-show host. Add these "personal" diet programs to the many medically endorsed and highly commercial diets already available, and we are bound to get confused.

In fact, we are so confused that it seems we often mix and match our plans according to our mood, and then change diets to suit us or our situation. Of course, this is to be expected, but it doesn't lead to a successful relationship with food, nor is it likely to make us especially happy when confusion and indecision inevitably set in.

I have worked with many clients over the years who believe that happiness can be achieved by reaching the "right weight." They go so far as to let the number showing on their scale every morning dictate whether they have a good day or a bad one, and change their diet accordingly throughout the day. Perhaps the typical "daily diary" will give you an idea of their thought processes:

Mix-and-match dieting

MONDAY MARCH 8th

I don't see why dieting has to be so hard.
I think I am being too strict, that's all.

Breakfast
▸ Oatmeal with honey—organic, from New Zealand.
F-Plan diet

Snack
▸ Still hungry. Switched to Atkins diet and had a small
bag of Brazil nuts.

Lunch
▸ Baked potato, no butter, low-calorie baked beans.
(Switched to Weight Watchers. I must be good.)

Snack
▸ Tomato sandwich (Hay diet)

Dinner
▸ T-bone steak and then some cheese (back to Atkins)

Snack
▸ Tiramisu (Does this qualify as the Mediterranean diet?)
▸ After-dinner chocolate mints (I'll start the diet properly tomorrow.)

The average dieter has tried so many plans
that he or she becomes adept at categorizing
several differing ways of eating into different
diets. You can see how it's possible to slot
almost any food into one diet or another,
if that's what you want to do.

The all-or-nothing diet

Or perhaps this "all-or-nothing" approach to dieting sounds more familiar to you?

MONDAY MARCH 1st

Today is the day I am going to finally lose this disgusting fat. I can do this. I will do it. I will walk to work and burn off the calories by taking the stairs and not the elevator. I will restart my gym membership and go every day. This is the beginning of a whole new me.

Breakfast
▸ Low-calorie cereal and skim milk, black coffee with fat-free sweetener and small glass of grapefruit juice (not orange, because doesn't that have a higher GI?)

Snack
▸ A small apple and hot water with lemon. Nothing else all morning

Lunch
▸ Low-calorie sandwich and a diet cola

Snack
▸ A rye cracker, no spread. Green tea (no sugar)

Dinner
▸ Green salad with tuna (in spring water, not olive oil), dressing of lemon juice and a teaspoon of olive oil, black pepper, and organic rock salt

Felt light-headed and hungry all day, but I know it's working . . . calories consumed 1,100 (barely).

Unsurprisingly, the dieter can't keep this diet up. A few days later her diary looks quite different:

THURSDAY MARCH 4th

It's all gone horribly wrong, I am a fat pig and everyone knows it, but no one is telling me. What an idiot I was to think I could lose weight, why do I even try? I overslept, missed breakfast, the kids were late for school, I was late for work, my boss is driving me crazy, I have two reports to finish before the end of the week, it's Robert's birthday, and I am supposed to be making dinner for him.

Breakfast
▸ Small Danish pastry, very small, in fact, so had two. Large latte with two sugars

Snack
▸ Granola bar and large cappuccino with two sugars

Lunch
▸ Club sandwich with a few French fries

Snack
▸ Birthday cake (I had to, it would have been rude to say no). Glass of Champagne. Cake was left in the kitchen, so I picked at it a little—mainly the frosting.

Drinks
▸ Two glasses of red wine and a bowl of peanuts

Dinner
▸ Lasagne and garlic bread (only thing in the freezer, he likes it and it is his birthday, after all). Caramel fudge ice cream

Calories 3,200

Alcohol and chocolate
Our relationship with alcohol is probably as complicated as the one we have with food. From time to time I have to ask a client to abstain from alcohol for a couple of weeks. Most people seem to struggle with this far more than with any other food or drink that might be off-limits. It is not unusual for clients to pull out their diaries and negotiate a time to begin this abstinence, even though going without alcohol is an integral part of their program. This even applies to clients who have lived with debilitating symptoms, such as abdominal discomfort or bloating, for several years. Despite the fact that I offer a practical solution that requires them not to drink for just two weeks so that they can reap the benefits, more often than not it is their attachment to alcohol that makes them reluctant to start my program.

How relevant are the health benefits?
I have lost count of the times that I have heard a glass of red wine is good for you, but I question whether it is good for weight control. Wine is made from grapes, which, like any fruit or vegetable, contain antioxidants. These are substances that are reputed to have the ability to combat inflammation, some forms of cancer, and cardiovascular disease. Wine contains resveratrol, a potent antioxidant that is the subject of much research. So surely wine is good for us? This may well be the case, and there is a lot of research that supports the theory, but if you want to maintain a healthy weight does this really matter? My professional and personal experience tell me that the potential benefits of wine, which have become part of our collective belief (the shorthand for which is "wine is good for us"), help us to justify drinking wine and other alcohol simply because it suits us.

I realize that this seems unsympathetic, but I do think we should be more realistic about alcohol. When it comes to weight issues, whether it is avoiding excess weight gain or losing weight, the potential health benefits associated with drinking red wine are irrelevant. The problem is that we drink too much, and when we have had a couple of glasses of wine, we really don't care that much about other things that might usually bother us. After a couple of glasses of alcohol we tend to want salty or fatty food, and the alcohol makes us worry less about our weight goals.

"The ruin of every diet has been drink."
A. D.

I understand that drinking alcohol helps to ease social situations, and we use it to relax and ease our stress levels. But it's hard to have just one glass and stop, and there is a lot of social pressure to drink.

Aside from the fact that drinking alcohol makes you put on weight, there is the aftermath to consider. Even small amounts of alcohol can lead to poor sleep quality, fatigue, and an increased desire for caffeine and carbohydrates. In itself this isn't especially bad, but it can easily affect your food decisions the day after drinking, too. We all know what happens when we drink too much, but we still do it again and again, although hopefully not every night!

While you consider the true cost of alcohol and ponder whether it is worth it or not, let me ask you one simple question: if there was a food that made you feel as bad the following day as alcohol does, would you eat it?

Our relationship with chocolate
We have a similar relationship with chocolate, and our typical thought processes about justifying its health benefits are only slightly different:

Cocoa beans contain antioxidants . . . antioxidants are good for you . . . chocolate contains cocoa beans . . . chocolate is good for you.

It is true that dark chocolate and red wine are better for you than milk chocolate and white wine, but this doesn't make them "good." We justify eating dark chocolate and drinking red wine because we want to.

Exercise: too much, too little

The benefits of exercise are plentiful, as anyone who exercises on a regular basis will agree. So it's a very worthwhile investment of time and effort.

When it comes to managing our weight, exercise is invaluable, and while it is possible to control your weight without exercising, it's an awful lot harder because you must pay relentless attention to what you eat. Take a look at the benefits of exercise and you will see that it's an impressive list (which includes reduced blood pressure, lower cholesterol and improved sleep).

When we think of exercise and weight control, it is understandably tempting to want to exercise simply to lose weight. I think this is potentially dangerous territory. You will have read about our metabolism and blood glucose in section one, and it's the interaction between these two essential elements and exercise that is important. The benefit of exercise on the action and effectiveness of insulin and the long-term effects on our metabolism are where the true value of exercise lies in respect to weight loss.

When we think of exercise and weight control, it is understandably tempting to want to exercise simply to lose weight. I think this is potentially dangerous territory.

However, the popular press, media, and advertising have all affected the way we think about exercise. I can understand why anyone would want to buy into "a better body in six weeks" or "look great for the beach." This sort of lure is better for business than "get stronger bones for the future" or "increase high-density lipoprotein," isn't it? Therefore, exercise can become part of the shorthand that we associate with quick weight loss. As a result, I believe that we often throw ourselves into an exercise program with the same "quick-fix" attitude that we adopt when we start a new diet. Because weight loss is such a huge source of potential revenue, gyms, swimming pools, and leisure centers have all resorted to using it to promote their services.

The kinds of phrases commonly used to promote these venues:

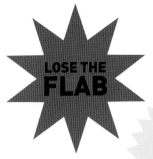

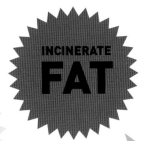

SHED THOSE UNSIGHTLY POUNDS

BURN CALORIES

While exercising may help with the process of weight loss, this type of terminology suggests a promise that is compelling yet misleading, and certainly promotes the "instant results" approach that I don't feel benefits our thinking.

When the exercise regime slips away

In addition, we try to factor exercise into our lives with such gusto that we are bound to have to cut back after a short amount of time. Gyms know all about this, which is why they market themselves in January to coincide with the "new year, new you" drive that we see every year. Go to any gym in January and it's likely to be busier than ever, yet by February the numbers are starting to drop off. Membership figures suggest that less than two-thirds of members make it through the first year, and that of the "January joiners" only a quarter will still be attending by the end of the year. It doesn't really matter when you join, as I believe that we set ourselves the same sort of unachievable goals that we do with our weight loss. It's not unusual to start an exercise regime aiming to fit something in most days, and when you are in the early stages it feels wonderful, as the endorphins kick in and improve your mood. We lose a few pounds and it seems like the answer to everything.

However, this approach to exercising, while admirable, simply isn't sustainable, and when something gets in the way—and it will—of the time you have put aside to keep fit, then you let the exercise routine slip away. I have found that when this happens a familiar sense of failure can creep in, which is when we can all too easily slip into the "Why bother?" mode of self-sabotage. Typically, you may find that a newly inspired dieter decides to exercise three or four times a week and follow all the advice that the health and lifestyle magazines espouse, such as fitting exercise into your schedule as if it were an appointment, and even hiring a personal trainer to get you into the right frame of mind. If four times a week in the gym or at the pool is worthwhile, affordable, and manageable, that's fine, but our natural enthusiasm and the tendency that many of us have to drive ourselves often mean that we take on too much. Our thinking may go something like this:

"I am so unfit, I have to do it. I am going to exercise every morning."

But when real life takes over and you miss a couple of days due to commitments or fatigue, your thinking changes.

"I have missed a couple of days, but no matter: I shall start again at the end of the week."

Or, and I fear that this is more likely, you might think,

"I knew I would fail. Why did I even think that I could keep this up? My trainer is going to be annoyed, but I will start again next week. In the meantime ..."

What can happen at this point is that if we think that exercise is a manifestation of being "good," when our routine stops or is interrupted, our eating patterns go the same way. My experience of this situation is that once the exercising lapses, poor eating habits creep back in.

Too much exercise

Can there be such a thing? Surely, if exercise is so good for you, then lots of exercise is even better? Well, up to a point this is true, but it depends on the individual's character.

If we use exercise as a reason to overeat, justifying what we eat by believing that we will burn it off in the gym the next day, we are playing a risky strategy. Creating a large deficit between energy intake and expenditure, whether through undereating or over-exercising, can have a detrimental effect on the metabolism. While eating too few calories is perhaps the worse of these two extremes, exercising too much isn't far behind. The trick is to be consistent, as we will see in section three.

The cost of a diet

One aspect of the cycle of dieting and overeating that I think we often overlook is cost. It's not the emotional cost I am talking about—that's something we look at in far more detail elsewhere in this section. This is the financial cost to you of losing and gaining weight. If you have never dieted before, the emotional cost may be hard to appreciate, but when it comes to how much a diet hurts your pocket, well, perhaps that's easier to relate to.

Diet foods and groups

When people feel they should be losing weight, they are likely to follow the most popular ways to do so, and I think it's fair to say that the best-known methods for losing weight are those that have been around for a while and are also the most highly marketed. The theory is that the cost of joining a diet group, for example, is minimal, although it can become pricey when you go every week. The cost also soon mounts up if you choose to eat a particular brand of low-calorie food, although the outlay—in theory—shouldn't add up to much more than you might spend on food anyway. The claim of your preferred diet plan is that, if you stick to it closely, all the plan will cost you is the weekly fees and the optional food.

However, I know from experience that most people don't stop there. Once the cycle of dieting has begun, there are other costs to take into consideration.

Clothing

You may want to try this easy experiment, which helps to give a further idea of the finances involved in dieting. Go to your closet and pick out the ten or so items of clothing that you wear most often, together with five more that you save for special occasions. They may be very formal, or slinky and glamorous; you choose. Estimate how much they cost to buy, repair, dry-clean, and store.

Now double that figure, and then triple it.

The cost of dieting should take into account the cost of the clothes that you can wear when you are at your slimmest, and then a second set for when you let things go a little. You may also want to factor in a third set, which are the clothes that you have to wear when weight loss eludes you. Just in case you are thinking that the third set is the sort you see in the "after" shot on a weight-loss advertisement, where a now-slim man stands inside his old trousers and pulls the waistband out to show how much he has lost, that third set doesn't have to be that much bigger than your second set of "normal" clothes. So for a woman, the sizes need only range from an 8 to a 12 or 14, and for a man, the difference between a 32-inch and 36-inch waist. That fluctuation of weight gain or loss is all that is needed to make more clothes a requirement (see also Fat clothes, thin clothes, pp.124–25).

The cost of dieting should take into account the cost of the clothes that you can wear when you are at your slimmest, and then a second set for when you let things go a little. You may also want to factor in a third set for when weight loss eludes you.

Exercise

Aside from your regular clothing, there is your exercise gear. Obviously we should all be exercising regularly, but on top of the various sizes of day-to-day clothes you may now have, you may also want to factor in the cost of exercise clothes in varying sizes, too. Added to which, if you are overweight, you are more likely to spend money on exercise equipment than someone who is a "normal" weight. Such equipment includes those advertised by flat-stomached models who create the illusion that their enviable bodies were honed by simply using the equipment that is being advertised. If you are overweight and fed up about it, these kinds of ads are probably going to appeal to you. Even the brightest of people can be taken in by such promises, and these machines aren't cheap. I have been told by ex-executives of television shopping channels that the majority of exercise machines are either never used or are used, on average, no more than a total of three times by the purchaser.

Professionals

Many people who are overweight spend money on personal trainers. On the surface this seems like a healthy thing to do, but I have worked with countless people over the years who embark on an exercise regime alongside a strict diet, which does, of course, result in weight loss. But then the diet is allowed to slip a little, as is the exercise, and the cycle starts again.

I do believe that an awful lot of money is spent trying to find a reason why people can't lose weight, when much of it is due to the repeated cycle of dieting in the first place.

Other professionals who might be employed are nutritionists, chefs providing personal cooking services, and health professionals. The latter are consulted in the hope that there is something medically wrong with the individual that might cause the excess weight. Of course, this may well be the case and I am not unsympathetic to this type of situation, but I do believe that an awful lot of money is spent trying to find a reason why people can't lose weight, when much of it is due to the repeated cycle of dieting in the first place.

Lastly, there is the cost of searching for a possible food allergy, which can also become very expensive and is mostly fruitless. It's a sad truth that many people seem actually to want to have a food allergy or intolerance that might explain the cause of their weight issues. In fact, many of the companies that market and sell allergy tests link the possibility of positive results to potential weight loss which, needless to say, we are often taken in by. After all, wouldn't it be marvelous if our weight gain wasn't caused by our lack of education and understanding about food, avoidance of exercise, or even simply our overeating, but was the fault of a food that we could then avoid?

"Other than my mortgage, I have spent more money on losing weight than anything else."

H. T.

"Being overweight has dominated my life. It's the one thing anyone would say about me if they were asked to describe me and sometimes I fear that's all they see: a fat woman."

M. L.

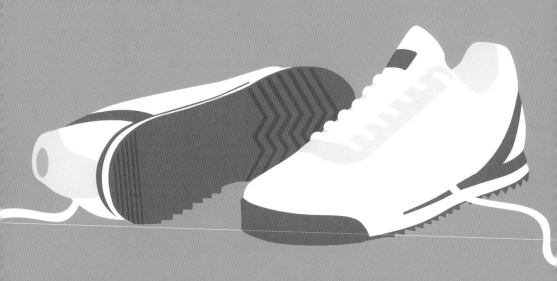

Coping with the pace of a diet Several years

ago I remember seeing a documentary on television about diets, in which a number of women each undertook a different diet; the results were then compared. Since diets are judged on their results, the "winning" diet was deemed to be the one that delivered the most weight loss in the shortest period of time. I remember that the winning diet was a very low-calorie diet. I also remember thinking that whoever had undertaken it would be paying the price with hunger throughout the diet, and the negative affects on her metabolic rate would contribute to problems in the future.

The reality of dieting is that we do want, albeit secretly and quietly perhaps, for the diet we follow to be one with spectacular results that can be achieved in a very short space of time. However, diets don't work that way, or at least not in the real world.

Many people embark upon a diet in advance of a big event, such as a family celebration or a vacation. Given that fast weight loss is just a promise away when you read a book or a feature in a magazine or newspaper, it's unlikely that, having booked two weeks in the sun for late July, you decide to start losing the weight in March. It just feels too far away; the trip isn't real yet. If it's a family event you are attending, the same thing happens. However, when it does start to feel real a month or so beforehand, the sense of panic takes over and we go for it. Our diet starts in earnest as we are motivated by the lack of time we feel we have.

If you or anyone you know has dieted, you may be familiar with the success that often occurs in the first week. When we cut our calorie intake in order to force the body to dip into its fat stores for energy, we are asking it to do something that it is reluctant to do.
The fat stores are there for the long term, and before they are given up, all the glycogen (p.25) has to be used up first. Since glycogen is held in a water base in the muscles and liver (and, to a lesser extent, in the tissues as well), in order to release it we inevitably lose water, too, which accounts for much of our weight loss in the first week or ten

days. We think it's fat being lost, but it's not, and that first week becomes the benchmark by which we gauge our progress. It is quite possible to lose 5 or 6 pounds in the first week (2–2.5 kg) and then after that things slow down, as the maximum fat that can be released is around 2 pounds per week (just under 1 kg). Given that your big event is just a month away, it is safe to say that you can't lose more than 10 or 12 pounds (4.5–5 kg) in the first month (which is pretty good going anyway).

We really need to understand the pace of a diet in order to be comfortable with our likely weight loss, but we also need to consider what effect it might have on us in the long term. If we leave things too late, we are more likely to go to extremes, either with food or with exercise or both in order to force the body to shed its weight. Weight loss aside, I do wonder what the emotional cost of dieting in this way is. Not just the extremes, but the pressure we put ourselves under when we try to lose weight in a given time frame. Surely this is a recipe for misery and hunger?

We really need to understand the pace of a diet in order to be comfortable with our likely weight loss, but we also need to consider what effect it might have on us in the long term. If we leave things too late, we are more likely to go to extremes, either with food or with exercise or both in order to force the body to shed its weight.

Weekly food diary

What follows is an example of what we might eat, thinking that we are doing the right thing to lose weight. While the food in this diary is low in calories, I imagine that our dieter will understandably be hungry for the early part of the week. But by the end of the week, he or she is fed up and compensates for the early abstinence by overeating. Although Monday's breakfast, for example, contains little fat and very few calories, it doesn't supply enough energy to fuel an average adult. This pattern is repeated in all the meals in the first few days, so it's no wonder that pizza and wine take on an alluring quality. This diet is, in effect, a seesaw diet because it veers from one extreme to the other.

"Dieting has ruled my life. It feels like I have spent a lifetime on a diet. I can't look at food without wondering if this is going to be the start, or the end, of yet another diet."

K. H.

MONDAY – START DIET

Breakfast
▸ Half a grapefruit, some low-fat cereal with skim milk, small black coffee

Lunch
▸ Low-fat sandwich and an apple

Tea time
▸ Granola bar, tea with skim milk. SO hungry

Dinner
▸ Stir-fried chicken strips with lots of vegetables. Roll on, bedtime.

TUESDAY

Breakfast
▸ Half a grapefruit, some low-fat cereal with skim milk, soft-boiled egg, small black coffee

Snack
▸ Two apples, green tea with sweetener

Lunch
▸ Soup and two rye crackers

7 p.m. Gym

Dinner
▸ One apple (not hungry)

WEDNESDAY

9 a.m. Pilates class

Lunch with colleagues
▸ Caesar salad without dressing and diet cola (no wine). Feel fantastic!

Dinner
▸ Soup with cheese on toast

THURSDAY

Breakfast
▸ Two flatbreads with cheese

Midmorning
▸ Need reward—regular cappuccino

Lunch
▸ Just salad

Dinner
▸ Emma's birthday. Too much red wine!

FRIDAY—need day off

Dinner
▸ Pizza, red wine, garlic bread, ice cream Start diet again next week

Compliments, shame, and self-esteem

Being on a diet means different things to different people. For some people, it simply means being careful of what they eat and reining themselves in again if they overeat on vacation or at a celebration. They understand how to eat so that they can enjoy wonderful food and drink and take advantage of the plentiful times in which we live. They know how to stop themselves from going over their upper weight limit and have found a practical way to exercise and stay healthy.

Sadly, such people are very much in the minority, and they generally haven't experienced what it is like to battle with cravings, gaining weight, and the personal disappointment that comes with dieting.

As we've discovered, the majority of people *have* been affected by the desire or compulsion to lose weight, and they are mostly unhappy with the way they look. If being slim, as I have already mentioned elsewhere, implies that you have few needs, are in control, and that life is good, then, conversely, being fat suggests that you are needy and out of control, and that life isn't working out for you. In other words, being fat is a physical manifestation of failure. While I don't think that any of this is true, I do think that, deep down, this is the way people feel about excess weight. One has to be very secure and grounded to have no feelings whatsoever about the issue of fat, as it has been demonized to such a degree that it denotes some level of moral failure in an individual.

When we lose the weight

Given all this, what happens to your self-esteem and confidence when you are on a diet? Firstly, being on a diet is seen as a good thing, and, similarly, losing weight is to be applauded; you are demonstrating that you have acknowledged your problem and are doing something about it. If being fat suggests a degree of self-indulgence and a lack of control, then it follows that losing weight means some degree of denial and self-control. And so the process of losing weight is one that is generally supported by family, friends, and colleagues. Their positive nature is reinforced in several ways, and you may understandably relish the compliments you get. Comments such as "I can see it's all coming off" and "Aren't you good!" are cause for delight.

Here are some typical comments that a dieter is almost guaranteed to hear at some point.

1. Starting the diet:

"Good for you. I am sure you can do it."
"I admire you. I don't think I could manage it."

2. A week or so into the diet:

"Aren't you doing well!"
"I am sure you must be feeling so much better."
"I can really see it now, especially in your face."

3. Two weeks further into the diet:

"You look so different!"
"You look so much better!"
"Your skin looks so clear."
"Your eyes look so bright."
"You look ten years younger."

If you lose significant amounts of weight, those people who were supportive and full of compliments at the beginning may ease off a little. Although, pre-diet, the thought of being thin was really rather appealing to you, all you want now is to hear the ultimate Holy Grail of weight-loss compliments: "You want to be careful: you are beginning to look a little gaunt." Once you hear these words, you will know that your weight loss has resulted in complete success. Subconsciously, though, you now start thinking that you can be less strict about what you eat.

When we fall off the wagon

I have been "good" all week.
I have resisted the urge to overeat . . .
I have been to the gym, I have exercised . . .
I have walked the dog so often that the poor
thing is starting to hide from me in the
mornings . . .
I have said "No" to birthday cake. Twice . . .
I have started drinking more water . . .
I am enjoying hearing people tell me that
I look well . . .
I am enjoying losing weight . . .

So why do we mess it up? The week has gone well, and you feel
that you are used to the diet and it's really not that bad. You take
a moment to wander into the coffee shop and you have every
intention of getting a cup of green tea and a banana.

You wait patiently in line, trying not to pay too much attention to the
display of pastries as you shuffle forward, getting nearer the front of
the line. The barista leans into the display right in front of where you
are standing and takes a slice of rich, dark, moist chocolate cake,
places it in a bag, and hands it to the slim man or woman ahead of
you, along with a cappuccino. You watch as he or she sprinkles
chocolate over the white cloud of foamy milk.

But no, you don't need that, you are happy with your
green tea and the piece of fruit . . .

But then you have been good all week …

No, no, must be strong.

Your turn comes, and the smiling barista asks what you want and you open your mouth and find yourself ordering a slice of chocolate cake and a double mocha cappuccino. With whipped cream.

It tastes like nectar, every mouthful dances on your tongue as the warm, chocolatey coffee washes it down.

Do you stop there?

Well, now you have ruined it you may as well carry on and see just how much you can eat because after this you are REALLY going to have to diet to make up for it.

The weekend comes and you have a full breakfast with bacon and eggs. On both days. You go to the movies and eat popcorn AND a bag of candy. You meet friends for drinks, and, along with the three glasses of red wine, you eat the peanuts and the potato chips. You round it off with a curry takeout on Sunday night.

When we gain the weight back

So when you gain the weight back after having lost it on a diet, or even gain weight for the first time, this is what you might hear from the people around you:

"   **"**

Nothing. Silence. You are unlikely to hear anything, or at least no one will say anything to your face. Since losing weight is a good thing, it's a reason for celebration, support, encouragement, and praise. Gaining weight is a source of shame and a sign of failure; therefore, in our society, it is considered to be inappropriate to say any of the following:

That's a pity, after all your hard work.

I can see it is all coming back.

Your eyes are looking dull.

Your skin isn't as clear as it was.

You are looking older again.

I see you are wearing your baggy clothes again.

Oh well, I knew you couldn't keep it up.

These phrases make me feel slightly uncomfortable, and if you feel the same, this demonstrates yet again how becoming fat, or even growing bigger, is deemed to be wrong, "a bad thing" that perpetuates low self-esteem.

If you are reading this and you are a normal weight, ask someone who has lost and gained weight in the past if they relate to any of the statements here. There is a very high chance that they have heard most of them themselves. While you are at it, ask yourself if you have ever paid anyone a compliment when they have lost weight, and if you said anything when they gained it back? While you and I might not have particularly noticed their weight gain— and even if we did, it's certainly not a big deal for us—for the successful dieter who has basked in the attention and feeling of superiority that losing weight brings, this is a risky time. They are bored with the diet; and, having denied themselves for so long, what better reward than to eat? In this way food becomes the sin and the reward, the pleasure and the pain. Any weight gain represents failure and shame and often leads to panic or indulgence. Panic involves going back on the diet, which removes any choice for the dieter of what and how to eat. The boundaries that another diet imposes (and it doesn't matter which diet it is) bring a welcome template to the potentially out-of-control dieter. Indulgence, however, is the path to ruin—until the next diet, that is. Flushed with success and feeling vital and slim, the dieter slowly puts on weight, a little here, some there, and since no one says anything, they fool themselves into thinking that they are getting away with it. And anyway, "I don't want to look gaunt, do I?"

Food becomes the sin and the reward,
the pleasure and the pain.

Fat clothes, thin clothes

As we discovered in section one, from the neck downward our bodies are like machines responding to the countless triggers that influence them. The body can adapt to varying temperatures, levels of activity or rest, and intakes of food in a nonjudgemental and coldhearted manner. In other words, our highly evolved and sophisticated metabolism and the way in which food is broken down, glucose extracted, and energy created, carry no emotional value for your body, and neither does your body care that you think you could, or should, be slimmer.

Your body doesn't know that you overate last night because you deserved it, or that it was a reward for having worked hard through the week, or even because it was your birthday, despite the fact that your emotional thought processes might be entirely justifiable:

It's been a long week and I haven't had a chance to see many friends or family. I was only out on Tuesday evening and that was just to see a movie ... I have been good all week, worked hard, and done some exercise, and it's not easy to get to the gym ... anyway, who cares? It was Friday night and so a few of us met for some drinks and then we had dinner. I know I drank a little too much and I know I ate too much, but it's OK, as I deserved it ... Anyway, I can work it off at the gym today ... if I get there. I can always go tomorrow.

Does any of that sound familiar?

Suppose you didn't manage to get to the gym or take that long walk to make up for your excesses of Friday night, however "deserved" they may have been. It's probable that because you are in a period of not being quite as "good" as you might ideally like to be, you continue to eat and drink a little more, partly because you know that soon you will have to get back on track and get healthy. Again.

The following weekend you might be heading out to visit your family, and you find that your favorite pair of black pants—the ones that you wish you had bought two pairs of, as they fit really well and make you look slim and tall—are tight when you put them on, and you don't feel comfortable. Reluctantly, you change into the other black pants, which are part of your "fat wardrobe."

Many dieters rely on their own barometer to gauge their weight gain, and how clothes feel is often the most pressing reminder of size. You may know this sense of frustration and disappointment, and unless you are a relaxed person, this sort of situation is bound to cause you anxiety. In turn, anxiety takes you into a whole realm of self-doubt and low self-esteem, and is nearly always damaging.

Instead of being able to fit into those wonderful black pants, you must wear loose-fitting clothes—a reminder of your failure. And so, in an effort to get back into the pants you reluctantly go back on the diet with no more treats; from now on, it's low-fat food and no alcohol. You cancel plans with friends you would normally drink with. Perhaps you start to rise a little earlier than before to get to the gym before work; and, mercifully, the weight starts to disappear again. You are working hard at losing weight, and you feel released from the burden of self-loathing that started to creep into your daily thoughts.

But then what?

You can't manage the gym every morning, and you can't avoid the friends forever. In time, you inevitably slip and the cycle starts again and the black pants are put away in favor of the ones that are slightly more forgiving—at least until you can bear to go back on a diet. If you don't recognize yourself in this, I guarantee that you know someone, and probably several people, who do live like this, and such simple tasks can be a minefield for them.

An endless cycle of boom and bust?

Whether you are slim, thin, fat, chubby, or overweight, there are times of the year and times in our lives when we are likely to eat more and thus gain weight. Traditionally these are annual events, the most notable being Thanksgiving, Christmas, and New Year's and also our own summer vacations, especially those taken in the sun.

This cycle of boom and bust, feast and famine appears to be completely normal and unquestioned, yet this way of eating affects the metabolic rate in a way that contributes to weight problems in the long run. I doubt that anyone who is in their forties, for example, and finding that losing weight wasn't as easy as it used to be, realizes that their plight is as much linked to that January detox they did five years ago as it is to the mince pie they ate last week. Yet it's true.

It doesn't have to be that way, as I maintain that we allow it to happen simply because it's what we are used to. Furthermore, gaining weight at certain times of the year is so deeply ingrained into our psyche because the media coverage actively encourages it, and then offers the remedy shortly afterward. The most obvious example is the winter holiday season: Thanksgiving, Christmas, and New Year's Eve. Late November and December feel completely different from January, which seems far in the future while we are indulging ourselves—as we are encouraged to do. How does it feel to think that your long-term weight issues—all that anguish and effort—have been caused, not just because you ate too much, but simply because you allowed yourself to fall for the media influences of the day? In other words, this uncomfortable situation is not your fault, which you probably weren't aware of; but you can do something about it.

Go on, you deserve it

Just for a moment, pretend it's mid-December and every magazine, newspaper, and lifestyle television is devoted to the indulgence and celebration of December festivities. It doesn't matter what religion you are, or where in the world you live, or even whether you celebrate Christmas or not; because December is the last month of the year, and there is bound to be some sort of celebration or event to mark the passing of the old year. Office parties, catching up with friends and family, and general overindulgence are as much part of the December experience as Santa and mince pie.

Perhaps you are at home one evening, the television is on, and an advertisement for an upscale food store shows an image of a rich chocolate pudding slowly oozing indulgent dark cocoa sauce as a gleaming spoon pierces the yielding sponge to a soundtrack of seductive chill-out music. The next commercial is for a clothing store, and you see images of glamorous clothes in rich colors modeled by beautiful people as they greet one another at parties with enthusiastic smiles. Imagine what you might think if the next ad was for a chain of gyms complete with images of toned people grinning through an exercise class as the upbeat and energetic voiceover encourages you to join the gym to work off your flab.
It feels out of place; it shouldn't be there, should it? And how would the commercial for the chocolate pudding go down in mid-January? Wouldn't it seem equally out of place?

By the same token, December newspapers are filled with features on how to make a splash this Christmas, while the January features focus on weight loss and detoxifying your life, body, and mind. Do you see how the mood of the moment—in this case, two consecutive months—could affect how you eat? It doesn't really seem like a big deal, does it? But as you will know from reading about our metabolic rate in section one, the increase in calories that accompanies December indulgences influences the way our body works, as does the January diet.

Vacations
Things work the other way around when it comes to vacations: you pay the price before indulging yourself on vacation. Advertising and newspaper features focus on the appeal of your losing weight beforehand, as being seen in a bathing suit or swimming trunks is the ultimate confidence test. The unspoken subtext to this is that you cannot expose your pale flesh on the beach or by the pool if you are fat, and such shame must be avoided by dieting. You cut down on your

food, watch what you eat, and try to be as active as possible to lose a couple of inches around your waist and on your thighs. And of course it works—all diets do. So you arrive at your vacation spot feeling as if you are justified in belonging there, now that you have lost some weight. There is an amusing aspect to this, for the strangers on the beach or by the pool have no idea how you looked a few weeks ago, and short of your showing them a photograph (as in a before-and-after ad for a weight-loss system) they really aren't going to know quite how well you have done!

But now it's vacation time, and after all the stress of dieting you deserve to enjoy every moment of your break. Having denied yourself the pleasure of eating and drinking anything you wanted over the last few weeks just so you weren't laughed off the beach, what do you do? You eat. And drink. A lazy breakfast with that second muffin, a cup of coffee and a pastry as you explore the local town, or an ice cream after dinner as you walk by the beach, perhaps a few glasses of wine with lunch, or maybe a cocktail or two watching the sun set over the bay. It sounds lovely, and isn't that just what vacations are all about? Wearing your swimsuit and loose, floaty clothing draws your attention away from your inevitable weight gain. This is something that most people succumb to, and although it doesn't really matter, as your relaxation and enjoyment are, of course, more important than a few pounds gained, you do begin to think at the back of your mind that you can lose them again when you get home.

At the end of the trip you get back into your travel clothes, and whereas the jeans you wore on the outward-bound flight two weeks ago felt a little loose, now they are tight and you don't feel comfortable. You get home and go back to your normal life and your normal food routine and the weight comes off little by little.

This is yet another familiar example of the boom or bust, feast or famine cycle that forces your metabolism to adjust itself, first one way, and then another, leading to a slowdown in the long term, which leads to weight gain. And when we gain weight, what do we do? Go on a diet, of course. If you have lost just a few pounds before your trip and gained the same back over a couple of weeks, it's unlikely that there will be much of a problem, but there will still be some price to pay in time, even if it's just a little. The more your weight fluctuates, the more pronounced the problem becomes in time. The question I have to ask, as it becomes increasingly hard to manage our weight as we get older, is "Was that indulgence worth it?" At the time it felt great, there seemed to be no cost whatsoever, yet in the long term the cycle of feast and famine, demonstrated here by Christmas and summer vacations, directly contributes to our weight gain in the long term. I wonder how many of us truly understand this as we eat and diet?

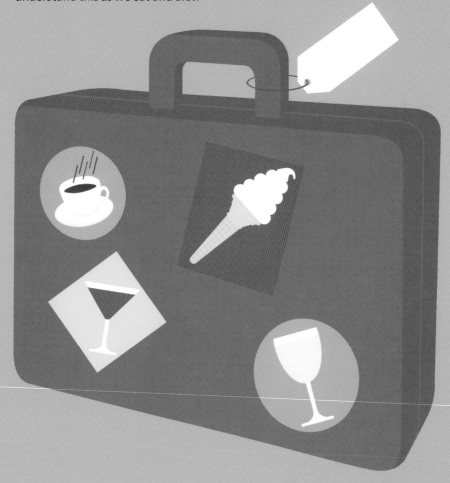

SECTION THREE
HOW TO EAT
SO YOU NEVER
HAVE TO DIET

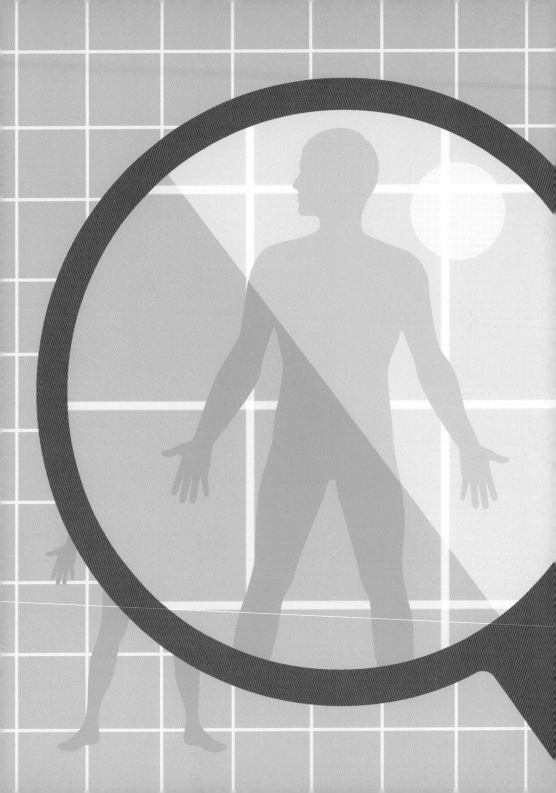

Over the past decade, I have come to believe that the weight problems many of us have are attributable to the fact that we don't know how to eat appropriately. As we've discovered, we know how to diet, and so eating as if we are constantly on a diet has become normal even for those of us who don't have a weight problem. This doesn't mean that we are all always on some rigorous fad diet, but we eat fearfully, as if we are really fat and food is the enemy that has to be conquered. I am sure that this attitude affects the way we approach the whole issue of eating, and in turn leads to weight gain over time.

Having explored the basic biochemical processes involved in the body's gaining weight (section one), and the multitude of factors that shape and influence our feelings and behavior toward food (section two), I am sure that you can see how our thought processes are often at odds with how we are built. Now it's time to learn how to eat in a way that promotes good health without your body laying down excess fat.

Let me make a couple of things clear at the outset of this section. This plan is not a diet; it is a way of eating that has several major benefits, including managing hunger and energy while still being able to enjoy food and eat well. It will not alert the metabolic rate to potential famine, which can lead it to slow down, nor will it encourage glucose to be stored away in the body as fat instead of being used to make energy.

This plan will not make you thin, but it will help you to maintain a healthy and natural weight that is appropriate for you. Despite the media pressure and images of skinny models, we know that the "ideal" body shape they promote is unnatural and unattractive, and not something we must aspire to. This plan is the antithesis of dieting, skinny, or thin.

Research tells us that factors such as eating alone or with strangers, not watching television (especially when eating), and not following one diet after the other can help us to eat less. Coming from a family that is genetically slim helps, too. Obviously we can't choose our parents, and eating alone or with strangers is not the route to happiness and healthy eating. However, we can choose not to follow diets, and I am confident that by applying my guidelines to how and what you eat, you can become immune to the lure of diets, diet foods, pills, supplements, tricks, and tips, so that they all fade into the background like white noise.

So the essential difference about my plan is that it is not a diet, and it should enable you to strip away all the confusing fuss around diets. I hope that once you have learned how to eat and not become fat you will be able to see that this plan is not something that you start, finish, come off, break, ruin, or stick to. It's something that you choose to keep on doing.

What to expect

My approach is not a diet, although it does most often result in weight loss. The difference between this plan and a diet is that a diet is something you embark upon with all the expectations and complications that we explored in section two. Diets have a beginning, a middle, and an end; my eating plan doesn't. If you understand my plan properly, you need never have to decide to go on a diet, postpone it, start it and fail, come off it, have a bad day, overeat at the end of it, worry about keeping the weight off, wonder if you should try another diet … I hope you get the idea.

All you have to do is follow the simple guidelines laid out in this section. My guidelines explain how you can create your own eating plan that is entirely in tune with the way your body functions, not at odds with it (like diets).

I do want to mention, once again, that if you are reading this book in order to lose weight, it is vital that you not see this eating plan as a "diet." If you do, you risk falling into the familiar and repetitive diet cycle that you may have seen other people succumb to again and again. This may even be something that you have done yourself, in which case here is a chance to end the cycle.

My guidelines explain how you can create your own eating plan that is entirely in tune with the way your body functions, not at odds with it (like diets).

The benefits of my plan

During the day our energy levels rise and fall, and are influenced by several factors: glucose levels in the blood, epinephine response, exercise, and quality of sleep. When our blood-glucose levels are low we are likely to feel hungry, and when hunger rears its confusing head, all those what-to-eat and diet thoughts are likely to surface.

If you eat in the way that I suggest, you will be able to keep your energy levels more consistent, which will help you to avoid worrying about being hungry and thus help you to avoid potentially confusing and self-sabotaging thoughts.

Rather than your having to exert willpower over what starts as a slight hunger pang and ends in a full-blown craving, my plan regulates your blood-glucose and energy levels, and therefore reduces your hunger pangs and the likelihood of cravings. It removes the desire to overeat or eat foods that you know won't serve you well (such as refined sugar and simple carbohydrates), so you don't have to get to the stage of fighting any cravings.

If you understand this aspect of my eating plan and apply it to your daily life, you can expect the following benefits:
- Your energy levels become more even and consistent
- Your hunger is manageable
- Cravings diminish

As we've established, on my plan you will be eating in a way that intelligently manages your glucose levels, which will lead to an even and consistent concentration of glucose in the blood.

In turn, this allows the body's cells to absorb the glucose made from food without overwhelming the cell. Therefore, the available supply of glucose equals the demand by the cell for fuel to convert into energy. In other words, you will make glucose at a consistent pace that feeds through to the cells in an easy forward motion without its bottlenecking (pp. 24–25).

By managing your glucose levels in this way, it is possible for you to manage your insulin levels accordingly. Bear in mind that insulin is released into the blood when glucose is present. By not allowing glucose to become too concentrated in the blood, insulin can fulfill its first role of encouraging the glucose into each cell, so that there isn't much excess glucose left lurking around the cells. As a result, insulin's second role of sweeping away any excess glucose to be stored temporarily in the liver is much more limited.

So another important benefit of my plan is that you won't be hurtling from feast to famine, dieting to overeating, being "good" and then ruining it all.

If you follow the guidelines of my plan and eat consistently instead of erratically, your metabolism will not be forced into "famine" mode, and it won't try to slow itself down to meet the reduced food intake that is inevitable when you are on a diet.

In other words, keeping your income regular and consistent establishes financial control and keeps you out of trouble. Your metabolism won't try to slow itself down if you follow my plan, and in the long run this should avoid the sort of weight gain that we associate with increasing age. Remember, if we have a slower metabolism, it means that we gain weight more easily, which then becomes increasingly difficult to lose and can exacerbate the cycle of dieting.

So the results of following my plan will be:
- Balanced glucose levels in your bloodstream
- Minimized insulin requirements by your body
- No interference to your metabolic rate

Is it really that simple?
Well, yes, it is, or at least it can be. It is my firm belief that the issue of diet, weight loss, and weight gain has become complicated and muddled to such a degree that is almost impossible for many of us to think clearly about it. In fact, if you followed even a third of the available diet advice that is thought to be "worthwhile," my guess

is that you would probably be changing diets every few days, with each diet program directly at odds with the previous one. Over the years, we have all been influenced by countless sources when it comes to diet and health, and while we know that many of the facts are useful and appropriate, much of what we have heard is either not true or not correct. It is up to us to try to filter all this information and consider exactly what the best course of action is.

There is no drama attached to this method of eating, just a regular intake of food. There is also no pain or deprivation, which is a good thing. If you feel that you need to lose weight, be prepared for slow and consistent results—again with no drama. This approach isn't easy for everyone, as many of us quite like the drama and pain associated with diets because we feel that this helps us gauge a degree of success. But by now you will be aware that such success is short-lived, and is inevitably followed by failure.

There is no drama attached to this method of eating, just a regular intake of food. There is also no pain or deprivation, which is a good thing. If you feel that you need to lose weight, be prepared for slow and consistent results— again with no drama.

In addition to understanding and following my approach, there is one more thing that you need to take into consideration. This plan suggests, for example, that you can choose to eat some nuts with a piece of fruit midmorning. If your first thought is, "Aren't nuts fattening?", you may want to consider how appropriate such thoughts are now and how they might continue to influence you to make poor food choices. Once you have learned to stop thinking in this way, you will know how to eat, not how to diet.

Where's my protein? In section one we explored the way in which the body digests three food groups. Just to remind you, carbohydrates are the easiest of the food groups to break down, and they provide glucose, which is the body's source of fuel. When we eat large amounts of carbohydrates, the glucose created can exceed the amount that is required by the cell to make energy. The cell is effectively flooded with glucose, and insulin has to sweep away excess glucose to be stored temporarily as glycogen.

Carbohydrates form the basis of most people's meals and snacks, as they are easily available, inexpensive, generally easy to prepare, and filling. When it comes to the food that we can buy when we are on the go, carbohydrates are again most prevalent, as they are the basis of most snacks and sandwiches. The ubiquitous coffee shops that are on every main street now are stacked with carbohydrate-based foods that appear to offer good value. It's worth remembering that carbohydrates create energy faster than any other food group; we do need them, as they also supply nutrients, fiber, bulk, and flavor. The problem is that most carbohydrate-based foods, such as sandwiches and pasta, contain comparatively little protein, so what we tend to eat is not as balanced as it could be if we want to eat for optimum health and regulated blood-glucose levels.

On the other hand, you may be familiar with high-protein diets that exclude carbohydrates and focus instead on eating mainly protein and fat. The initial success of these types of diet in helping you to lose weight occurs because the high amounts of protein that you have to consume forces the body into a state that is known as ketosis, in which fats are converted back into energy when glucose is lacking. In other words, if you eat mainly protein and consume no carbohydrates, your body is forced to give up its fat stores. However, you can't keep up eating in this unnatural way for very long, and your fat stores are inevitably refilled when you return to eating normally.

In section one we discovered that protein is broken down quite slowly by the body, and fat slower still, in comparison to how quickly carbohydrates are digested (p.29). So what you need to do to manage your hunger is actually very simple: combine the three food groups every time you eat. That means making sure that you eat some carbohydrate, protein, and fat for every breakfast, snack, and lunch every single day, week in, week out.

In reality, this might mean eating oatmeal or an egg and toast for breakfast instead of a low-calorie, grain-based cereal. If you have oatmeal, which is a complex carbohydrate, you must add some fat and protein to it, which means having a smaller portion of grain mixed with a generous palmful of slivered almonds and natural plain yogurt, for example. This breakfast will provide more calories than the low-calorie cereal, but oatmeal is made from whole oats, which take longer to be broken down into glucose. The almonds take even longer to be digested and also provide some fat, which is more satisfying to eat than just carbohydrates. In other words, this meal provides you with energy for far longer than the low-calorie option, and prevents you from feeling hungry for longer. It doesn't matter which protein you have, so you can be as maverick as you like—add chicken to your oatmeal, or tofu to cornflakes. You are free to combine any protein with any complex carbohydrate, and when you grasp this concept and apply it to your eating habits, you can be free forever from an endless cycle of dieting.

What you need to do to manage your hunger is actually very simple: combine the three food groups every time you eat. That means making sure that you eat some carbohydrate, protein, and fat for every breakfast, snack, and lunch every single day, week in, week out.

When it comes to dinner, the carbohydrates in grain-based foods (which are ideal for providing the body with energy during the day) are not so necessary in the evening, because we are unlikely to need as much energy at night. So for dinner we should forgo complex carbohydrates and eat the carbohydrates found in fresh fruits and vegetables with more protein to compensate (p.148).

Are there any other benefits? A little complex

carbohydrate combined with some protein and fat creates an ideal meal or snack that provides satisfaction on both a physiological and a psychological level for several reasons.

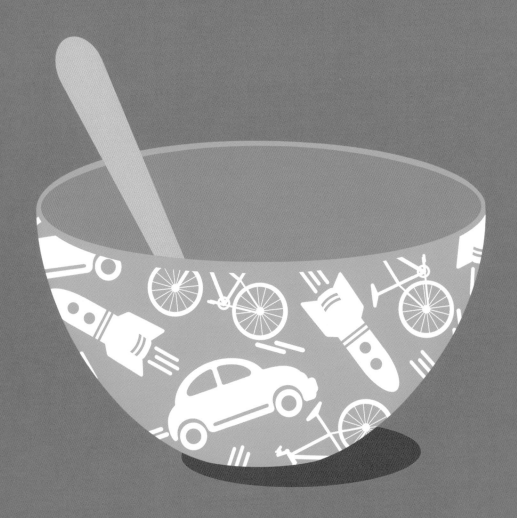

More energy

Combining the three food groups every time you eat encourages your glucose production to be consistent and relatively slow. Therefore, you will create enough energy for both the short and medium term. If you eat these food groups separately, your body's glucose levels become unbalanced: your energy levels soar briefly and then fall, which we often interpret as hunger. Either you eat again, which continues the cycle, or you battle not to eat, which makes you feel miserable and even more tired. So by making a significant difference to the way that glucose is created and used in your body, you will, in turn, be able to manage your energy levels so that you have more energy for longer. In doing so, your weight is also managed, as the glucose supply will be equal to demand and not in excess of it (which leads to glucose being laid down as fat rather than used to make energy).

By making a significant difference to the way that glucose is created and used in your body, you will, in turn, be able to manage your energy levels so that you have more energy for longer.

Textures, flavor, and the experience of eating

Eating should be a pleasurable experience and satisfy more than just your physical appetite. I am sure that you have experienced times when you have eaten dinner and found that although you might no longer be hungry, you still want to keep eating. There could be more than one reason why this might be so, but I believe that if what you eat satisfies more than just your hunger, the problem of overeating and grazing throughout the evening is far less likely to occur.

For example, you may decide to eat a simple food, such as plain yogurt. Although it contains some protein and carbohydrate, your experience of eating the yogurt on its own is probably, on the whole, bland and unfulfilling. However, if you add a chopped apple to the yogurt to include something with bite—a "crunch" element, if you like—you have to chew each mouthful to begin to break down the apple. By adding the piece of fruit, you have changed the eating experience. Take this one step further by adding some sesame seeds or slivered almonds, and compare the difference now.

You can now experience different ingredients and colors just by looking at the combined food groups in the bowl, and eating them together provides you with a variety of tastes and textures that have crunch, flavor, smoothness, and some fat, too (fat adds what the food industry calls "mouth feel," which is an essential part of the satisfaction of eating). This combination of food groups offers a more enjoyable eating experience, which should satisfy the appetite of both your mind and your body.

I believe that if what you eat satisfies more than just your hunger, the problem of overeating and grazing throughout the evening is far less likely to occur.

Hormones and satiety

I doubt that many of us consider hormones when we eat, but you may remember that in section one I mentioned two hormones that are associated with appetite—CCK (cholecytstokinin) and GIP (gastro-inhibitory peptide). When we eat fat, these hormones are released into the bloodstream. The first of these, CCK, is believed to reduce appetite, and GIP has a similar effect, albeit milder. While these hormones are not the "Holy Grail" of appetite control, they have a small effect in telling the brain that it has eaten and that all is well. So having some fat every time you eat is essential. This may also explain why low-fat diets are often associated with hunger, cravings, success and failure, and yo-yo dieting. Another hormone, leptin, which was first identified in the mid-90s, is also of significance. It, too, can reduce appetite, and there is some research to suggest that it can also stimulate the metabolic rate. When the concentration of leptin in the blood is normal, our appetite is satisfied. Leptin is the subject of extensive research at the moment, and I suspect that if a leptin-type drug is created it may be a huge leap forward in aiding weight control, although that possibility is still a long way off.

Combining the three food groups every time you eat encourages your glucose production to be consistent and relatively slow. Therefore, you will create enough energy for both the short and medium term.

Leptin is obviously not a substance that is found in any food, but early studies suggest that one food more than any other—fish—will favorably influence leptin levels in the body. It is the omega-3 fats found in fish that are believed to be of benefit. Populations that eat little or no fish have been found to have the lowest levels of leptin in the blood, while those that eat fish regularly have healthy levels. Although fish was the most significant of all the foods investigated in these studies, beans and legumes also have a beneficial effect, followed by vegetables and fruit.

The clear message that comes through from these studies may not be new—eat plenty of fish, beans, and fresh produce—but it does help to highlight *why* we should eat them, which can only be a good thing, especially if we combine them with the other food groups.

It is the omega-3 fats found in fish that are believed to be of benefit. Populations that eat little or no fish have been found to have the lowest levels of leptin in the blood, while those that eat fish regularly have healthy levels.

Eat little and often

The way to maintain a healthy weight is to eat, and eat regularly. We have already looked at the three food groups and how they should be combined for each meal or snack, and now we are going to add to that by looking more closely at how often you should eat.

As you now know, when eaten in the right proportions, the three food groups combine to create glucose that is released into the bloodstream at a slow and steady pace. This creates a situation in which the cells can absorb the glucose quite readily and are not overwhelmed by it (which then forces the excess glucose into storage). To remind you of the biological processes involved in digestion, here is the equation from section one that summarizes how the body produces energy:

FOOD ▸ ▸ ▸ GLUCOSE ▸ ▸ ▸ CIRCULATES IN BLOOD ▸ ▸ ▸ SURROUNDS AND ENTERS CELLS ▸ ▸ ▸ FUEL TO MAKE ENERGY
(BUT ANY EXCESS GLUCOSE THAT THE CELL CANNOT ABSORB IS SWEPT AWAY FOR STORAGE.)

The other important fact to note is how frequently you should eat, and you may be pleased to know that it is imperative that you do so often if you want to maintain optimum energy and manage your weight with confidence. In order to control your glucose levels effectively, you should eat every two-and-a-half to three hours; and, ideally, what you eat should be about the same amount every time. This challenges the old-fashioned idea that we should eat three square meals a day (although this traditional approach promotes a sense of "discipline" about eating, it doesn't actually get the best from the human body). Eating breakfast with the idea that it will "set you up for the day" or "see you through the morning" encourages you to eat more than your body can absorb and utilize, which then results in both glucose storage (as glycogen) and hunger pangs.

In practice, I believe that eating breakfast, a morning snack, lunch, an early afternoon snack, a late afternoon snack and then dinner—all of equal size, and mixing the food groups every time—is the ideal way in which to manage your glucose levels. Clearly this approach may not always fit in with your daily routine, but if you can make it work for your particular timings, you will be much better off because of it. I must stress that you won't be eating much more food than you would if you only ate three meals a day (you might even eat slightly less, as your appetite will be satiated more often), but your food intake will be apportioned differently.

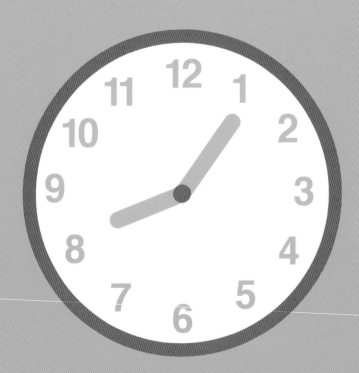

We will look at specific examples of meals on pages 150–52, but let's run through how this would work on a typical day. When you wake up, you should have breakfast within 30 minutes of rising, so if you get up at 7 a.m., eat breakfast at 7:30 a.m.

You should eat again two-and-a-half hours later, so that means that at 10 a.m. you can enjoy another mini-meal.

Lunch should then be at 12:30 p.m., followed by another small meal at 3:00 p.m. A last snack at 5:30 p.m. could precede dinner at 7 p.m.

It is quite possible that you will want to eat again at 9:30 p.m., but it is unlikely that this snack would be of the same quantity as the other meals that you will eat during the day (we will look at nighttime eating in more detail below).

How much do I eat?

If you are looking at this eating plan and you have a history of dieting, it is possible that you might find this concept of so many meals in one day a little daunting. Perhaps you don't trust yourself to eat this often for fear of overeating. Whether you feel this way or not, bear in mind that the important thing here is that although you will be eating often, it will be in smallish amounts.

While I am reluctant to suggest the exact amount of food you should eat, for fear of introducing an element of what could be termed "a diet" into this lifelong solution, it is really important to understand how much you should eat.

This simple exercise should make this issue very clear. Take a side plate (they do vary in size, but the standard size is 6 inches [15 cm]). Take a marker pen and use it to divide the circular plate into three equal-sized sections, as if you were dividing a pie into three equal pieces.

Perhaps you don't trust yourself to eat this often for fear of overeating. Whether you feel this way or not, bear in mind that the important thing here is that although you will be eating often, it will be in smallish amounts.

One of the sections will be for your protein. In another will sit your complex carbohydrates, and the last section is for vegetables or fruit. Obviously, you could eat more by simply piling the food as high as possible on the plate and while it is impossible to propose a height limit on your food, perhaps the best indicator is that the protein source should stand proud if you hold the plate at eye level. In other words, the fish or chicken—or whatever protein you have chosen— is the highest food on the plate. I hope that this visual gauge gives you a good indicator as to how much to eat without being too severe or prescriptive about your food. By now you will know that I firmly believe that we rebel at some point if we feel that we are "on a diet" and have to eat a restricted amount (and a limited variety) of food.

If you are wondering where the element of fat fits on this plate, it will either be contained in your protein (proteins are rarely fat-free), or perhaps added to the meal in the form of a little oil. Remember that you can have more than one protein, so long as the amount of each protein is still limited to the one-third portion. You might choose, for example, to reduce the size of, say, a piece of chicken breast or salmon steak and add some seeds, which will supply a "crunch" factor.

Remember that you can have more than one protein, as long as the amount of each protein is still limited to the one-third portion.

Day versus night

During the day you will be eating five times to supply you with enough energy for the ensuing hours. Therefore, those five small meals should all have the same ratio of protein to carbohydrates (which is one-third each).

In the evening things change a little, as our energy requirements are likely to be reduced before we go to sleep. So the proportion of carbohydrates to protein needs to change in favor of more protein on the plate. So instead of dividing your plate into three equal portions, you

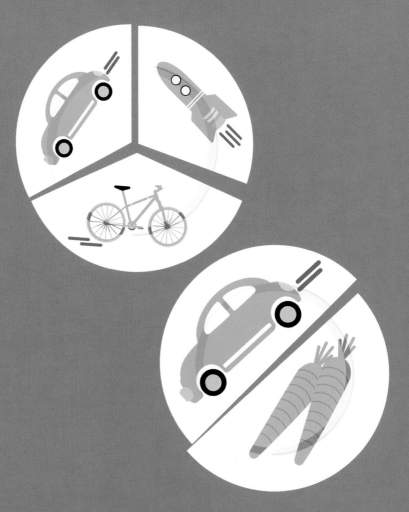

simply draw a line down the middle. Half of what you eat in the evening will be protein and the other half will be fresh vegetables or fruit.

The emphasis here should always be on vegetables, not fruit, simply because I believe that the more fruit you eat, the stronger your desire for sweet foods. Of course, you can eat fruit in place of sweetened foods, but fruit as a whole can come under the heading of "Surely it's better than . . . ?" (p.162).

But what if I'm not hungry?

The trick is to eat when your hunger is minimal and not "out of control." Your hunger is not there to be beaten, ignored, or conquered; instead, you should respond to it. A small amount of hunger is what you want to aim for. Many people find that when they eat with regular frequency, their hunger is greatly reduced at all times. However, there is a trap that you can fall into, and that is thinking that if you aren't too hungry, and it feels manageable, you can try to use this as a reason to skip a meal so that you eat less and cut your calorie intake. This approach won't work in the long term, as eating frequently is the real key to success.

Socializing

If your reaction to this concept of eating frequently is to wonder how you will manage it if you work in an office, or are always on the go, or you are going to eat out, you can easily overcome this potential difficulty by ensuring that you eat at times that work for you. Extending or reducing the period between meals a little here and there won't make a big difference between your being fat or slim in the long run, but if you know that you will have extended periods of time when you can't eat a meal, then you need to keep a snack on hand in your bag, knapsack, or car so that you will be able to eat something to keep your glucose levels consistent.

It is really important that you not skip any meals, and that if you do so for any reason, you not then overeat at the next meal to make up for it. From time to time you may well do both, but so long as you have a regular consistency in your usual routine of eating, the occasional variation shouldn't matter too much.

Typical meals
As you know, the issue that I have with diets is that, for one reason or another, they are too prescriptive, which means that failure is often inevitable and perpetuates an unhealthy cycle. So the meals that I suggest here are merely that—suggestions. They represent the typical foods that an adult might eat in a day, although these lists are not complete by any means.

The simple truth is that in order for the food you eat to benefit your mind and body, all three food groups need to be represented in each meal or snack, and your intake of food needs to be consistent in terms of both amount and frequency.

Sample breakfasts
- One or two scrambled, poached, or soft-boiled eggs with wholewheat or rye toast
- Live natural plain (not sugared) yogurt with chopped fresh fruits and sunflower and pumpkin seeds
- Oatmeal with live natural plain yogurt, chopped apple or banana, and any nuts, as long as they are plain (not sugared, honey-roasted, or salted)
- Smoothie made with live natural plain yogurt, pear, pumpkin seeds, sesame seeds, and a little apple juice. Blend until smooth
- Low-sugar granola with added fresh fruit and any nuts or seeds of your choice
- Rye toast with hummus
- Last night's salmon with flatbreads
- Cornflakes with roast beef

The truth is that ANY complex carbohydrate combined with ANY protein will do, so if you want cornflakes with roast beef, have it, even if it isn't the most traditional of ways to start the day.

Sample lunches

- Baked potato with baked beans (for protein) and a large mixed salad
- Soup made from vegetables and lentils or beans for a well-balanced protein/carbohydrate meal in a cup, or any soup, together with rye bread or soda bread
- Broiled tofu or egg with a large salad that contains at least five different vegetables and some crusty bread
- Caesar salad or goat cheese salad with flatbreads
- Omelet with vegetables, mushrooms, tomatoes, and some cold rice left over from last night's dinner
- Sandwich overfilled with chicken or tuna and lettuce and tomato

What about rice with chicken and peas? That will work. So will sardines with quinoa and fava beans. As will kidney beans with tomato and a slice of bread. Once again, any protein with any complex carbohydrate will do, so choose anything from the lists on pages 31 and 32 and combine it in any way that you want.

Remember: any protein, any complex carbohydrate

Sample dinners

- Broiled veal with two or three vegetables, including snow peas and green beans
- Stir-fried mixed vegetables including asparagus, mini corn, and carrots with your choice of protein
- Thai green curry with beans and vegetables
- Roasted Mediterranean vegetables with goat cheese, mozzarella, or feta cheese
- Large bowl of mixed vegetable soup with chicken, fish, kidney beans, or black-eyed peas
- Greek salad

Once again, these suggestions are merely that; add in some of your own choices to make sure that you are comfortable with this theory. Think about your favorite meal and see if it works; if not, what small changes could you make to adapt it and make it more suitable?

Sample midmorning and afternoon snacks

- Hummus on a flatbread with mixed raw vegetables such as carrots, celery, Belgian endive, beans
- Apple or pear with small piece of Cheddar or other hard cheese
- Handful of unsalted nuts or mixed seeds with a piece of fruit
- Almond, cashew, or peanut butter on rice cakes
- Cottage cheese on (sugar-free) corn cakes

Sample evening snacks

- Live natural plain yogurt with mixed seeds
- An apple and some Brazil nuts
- Hard cheese and sliced vegetables

"It feels like I am eating all the time—I never crave food and my hunger is manageable."

M. L. T.

"Can I really eat this much? It feels wonderful to be able to eat for a change."

K. H.

Sugar

Although I think that cutting out any food has several diet traps attached to it—namely that as soon as it is forbidden it becomes more tempting and desirable—my experience tells me that sugar is the one foodstuff that we need to watch out for. While fat has been consistently demonized due to its inherent calorie content, it could be argued that sugar has slipped quietly under the radar in the meantime.

We will look more closely at different types of sugar, but in essence they are all the same: they have been processed from sugarcane plants and are converted from food to glucose very rapidly by the body, which means that when we eat sugar we experience some noticeable fluctuations in blood glucose. Although this may not have much in the way of repercussions with regard to weight gain, this fluctuation will lead to hunger and cravings. In other words, sugar makes you desire more food, and often more sugar. At this point, you will slip into the realms of trying to control your cravings, and while you might manage a degree of self-control most of the time, you simply can't do it all the time. Furthermore, it's an unhappy situation, which you may know about already: cravings are the death knell of any diet. However, if you avoid sugar, you will greatly minimize any sweet cravings you might have and make it easy for you to enjoy the rest of your food.

When we eat sugar we experience some noticeable fluctuations in blood glucose.

Cane, brown, and organic sugar

While white sugar is the stuff that converts into glucose most quickly, other sugars, despite their aura, are not far behind. Yes, they are "better" than refined white sugar, but this doesn't make them "good." They fall into the "Surely it's better than …?" category , which we discuss on page 162.

Honey

Honey can be problematic; it is converted by the body from food to glucose at a slower speed than sugarcane, but this doesn't mean that it can be categorized as a food that is broken down slowly. It does fall into the "Surely it's better than ... ?" category, but it isn't as bad as brown, cane, and organic sugar. Honey does have beneficial qualities but these aren't properties that can't be found elsewhere, and eating honey simply makes the desire for sweet food more of an issue.

This isn't a deal breaker, but if you want long-term success in managing your weight and you want to make your life easy, stay away from sugar in all its forms (which includes artificial sugars, molasses, and corn syrup). If you do so, managing your blood glucose levels becomes an easy thing to do and will liberate you from sweet cravings.

If you want long-term success in managing your weight, and you want to make your life easy, stay away from sugar in all its forms.

The taste of sugar might be pleasurable, but it is a pleasure that will quickly diminish as you apply my plan. This does not mean that you can never eat sweet food again, but you shouldn't eat it regularly. You might feel like a couple of squares of dark chocolate (which is naturally low in sugar) after a meal, which is fine, as the presence of protein and fat in your meal will slow down the way that the sugar is broken down. Having more than two squares, however, will counteract the action of protein and fat and lead to fluctuations, cravings, desire, and weight gain ... you know how it goes.

If you have a "sweet tooth," turn to pages 162–63 for why we might need to remove this and several other phrases from our lives.

Alcohol

Alcohol is a really problematic issue, as it is ingrained in our society to such a degree that people who don't drink are considered to be unusual. On pages 104–05 we looked at some of the myths and social conditioning that we have probably all experienced about drinking. I also suggested that if there was a food that made us feel as bad as alcohol does, we probably wouldn't eat it. Think about it: If there was a food that changed your behavior for the worse, was full of calories, offered negligible nutrition, and made you gain weight due to the aftereffects of its chemicals, would you really eat it?

One of the problems with diets is that they inevitably restrict what we eat, which then leads to the risk of feeling deprived. I believe that a successful eating plan—one that you understand and can apply day in, day out—doesn't come with restrictions. Real long-term success lies in removing, not resisting, the desire for the sort of food that will lead to weight gain. With this in mind, how does alcohol fit in? The truth is that it doesn't really fit in at all. In other words, if you want to manage your weight for life, you shouldn't drink alcohol. Yet being a nondrinker brings with it a social pressure, as many people are uncomfortable with someone not drinking alcohol. I realize that this is not a popular option, and for those people who find that thought too extreme or unacceptable, there is a second way.

If you want to manage your weight for life, you shouldn't drink alcohol.

Some things to remember about alcohol are that, firstly, any food that is in the stomach will pass more quickly into the gastrointestinal tract in the presence of alcohol. By artificially speeding up the process of digestion, it is possible that the food will break down into glucose too rapidly, which will inevitably lead to insulin grabbing some excess glucose to store away. However, meals that contain a combination of fat, protein, and carbohydrates will be the least affected by this, so there is a way to drink some alcohol and minimize its ill effects.

However, if you have a few drinks, the following day is often a potential danger zone, as that's when you will feel slightly under par, which can lead to carbohydrate and caffeine cravings. Since this plan takes into account the overall influence of what we eat and drink, and not just the isolated effects, drinking alcohol can make it more difficult to exert willpower and resist tempting foods. You may win most of the time, but you won't all of the time. And when you don't, your intake of alcohol will increase, as will your taste for carbohydrates—and "hangover food" isn't going to do you any favors.

Drinking alcohol can make it more difficult to exert willpower and resist tempting foods. You may win most of the time, but you won't all of the time.

The compromise is to have one glass of wine with your main course from time to time. If you were hoping for better news, then I offer my apologies, but that's the reality of the problem. If you find yourself thinking along the lines of "But isn't red wine good for you?" or "But vodka is pure" or "No way am I having just one" then that is your decision; but in my opinion, that decision will make managing your weight that much more difficult.

I often tell clients who want to drink alcohol that they should limit their drinking to weekends and Wednesdays, which allows them to have days when they are not that far away from their next drink, but which should help to alleviate any feelings of deprivation.

If you have drinking buddies, or a group of friends with whom you always drink, then see them on one of the appointed days. If the point of being together is drinking, then you may wish to look again at why you do this, and whether it really benefits you.

There can be no doubt that alcohol serves many purposes, not least easing social situations, helping us to bond and relax, and so on. Its value to you may outweigh the importance of staying lean, or it may not, and that's a personal decision that only you can make.

Caffeine

There is nothing "wrong" with caffeine. I have no feelings about whether it is good or bad for you, but in the context of long-term weight management, I don't think that it should figure too often.

In section one we looked at how caffeine affects our digestion (pp.20-21). In short, caffeine leads to a short-term rise in energy levels, which is followed by a feeling of fatigue that can lead us to eat more. Furthermore, caffeine leads to fluctuations in energy levels, and having one cup of whatever-it-is simply leads to a desire to have another cup. Caffeine is unlikely to raise your glucose levels directly, but it will influence it indirectly in three ways. Firstly, by encouraging food to leave the stomach before it is fully digested, caffeine can speed up the way that glucose is made (admittedly, this is a minor link, but one we should be aware of). Secondly, caffeine can interfere with the action of insulin, which means that the glucose created from food does not enter the cell quite so readily, leaving it circulating around so that it is stored away instead. Thirdly, caffeine increases epinephrine levels, which in turn encourage glucose levels to rise.

Smoking

I am sure that all smokers know the enormous risk that they take with their health. Even if the dangers are not immediately apparent, there is no valid reason to keep smoking. I know that people who smoke are often afraid to stop, as they worry about possible weight gain; they usually choose to smoke a cigarette instead of eating. Indeed, many people actually start smoking in an effort to avoid overeating. I have worked with several clients who have stopped smoking and then successfully managed their weight by adopting the principles of this plan. If you are a smoker, there is no reason why this plan won't work for you, too, so I encourage you to quit smoking and follow the guidelines set out in this section.

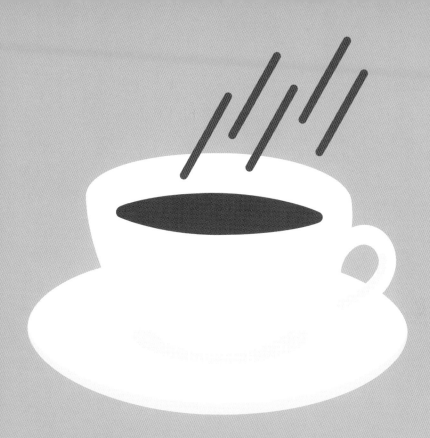

Caffeine, therefore, has an influence on weight gain. So, in the context of not putting on weight, and because caffeine has a potentially detrimental effect on our physiology as well as our psychology, I suggest that you not have caffeine.

Surely one cup can't hurt?

No, one cup is not going to hurt at all, and if you would like to have a cup of a caffeinated drink with breakfast or whenever, go right ahead. But in the context of avoiding weight gain for life, I suggest that you not have any. Switch to alternatives that are naturally free from caffeine, or have very little. These include green and white tea, and you can still drink decaffeinated regular tea or coffee.

What you can eat

barley, oatmeal, oat flakes, rye grain, wholewheat flour, white flour, wholewheat pasta, white pasta, wholegrain rice, white rice, red rice, couscous, chicken, turkey, quail, rabbit, partridge, pheasant, beef, lamb, ox, pork, ham, bacon, liver, kidneys, heart, cannellini beans, black beans, black-eyed peas, fava beans, kidney beans, lima beans, butter beans, pinto beans, haricot beans, shrimp, prawns, lobster, oyster, cockles, clams, mussels, scallops, squid, anchovy, bluefish, turbot, carp, cod, Dover sole, eel, flounder, gray mullet, haddock, hake, halibut, herring, lemon sole, mackerel, mahi mahi, marlin, monkfish, orange roughy, perch, pollack, rainbow trout, red mullet, river trout, salmon, sardines, sea bass, sea trout, shark, skate, swordfish, tuna, turbot, whiting, rice milk, coconut milk, skim milk, low-fat milk, whole milk, beer, spirits, wine, tofu, baked beans, duck eggs, hens' eggs, quails' eggs, soy milk, nut milk, low-fat yogurt, full-fat yogurt, Greek yogurt, low-fat cottage cheese, full-fat cottage cheese, cream cheese, goat cheese, feta cheese, low-fat cheese, full-fat hard cheese, full-fat soft cheese, butter, green lentils, yellow lentils, red lentils, brown lentils, edamame, quinoa, chickpeas, bananas, coconuts, pears, pineapple, plums, grapes, apples, nectarines, peaches, apricots, dates, strawberries, blueberries, blackberries, red currants, black currants, cranberries, loganberries, gooseberries, watermelon, cantaloupe melon, honeydew melon, starfruit, cherries, kiwi fruit, bananas, kumquats, mangoes, papayas, lychees, mandarin oranges, tangerines, grapefruit, clementines, oranges, lemons, limes, potatoes, broccoli, spinach, cabbage, kale, peas, brussels sprouts, artichokes, asparagus, beans, tomatoes, avocados, lettuce, Chinese cabbage, parsnips, turnips, cauliflower, squash, pumpkins, onions, garlic, celery, fennel, arugula, leeks, greens, bok choy, peppers, mushrooms, bean sprouts, eggplants, beets, carrots, celeriac, olives, zucchini, marrows, yams, sweet potatoes, sunflower oil, olive oil, canola oil, vegetable oil, avocado oil, pumpkin oil, sesame oil, sunflower oil, corn oil, hazelnut oil, walnut oil, Brazil nuts, almonds, hazelnuts, walnuts, macadamia nuts, pecans, peanuts, cashews, chestnuts, nut butters, pine nuts, linseeds, pumpkin seeds, sesame seeds, sunflower seeds, hemp seeds

What you can't eat

SUGAR

It's that simple: avoid sugar
in food products and on its own.

Surely it's better than...?

When people seek advice from a nutrition expert they will often ask about a specific food. I generally find that they are most interested in finding out whether something they like to eat is "good" or "bad." For example, if a client eats a lot of dried fruit and I suggest that they may be an unnecessary source of concentrated sugars, the client invariably responds by saying, "Surely it's better than having chocolate?" And yes, it *is* better than chocolate, although that doesn't make the food in question an ideal choice.

"Surely it's better than...?" is an expression often used by clients, and I find that it is usually applied to chocolate or red wine. Having dark chocolate is understandably justified by suggesting that it's better than having milk chocolate—and it is. Many clients justify drinking red wine by saying that it is better than white wine (simply because of the inherent antioxidant properties of the darker grapes from which it is made). From that perspective it is better than white wine.

I am not saying that you shouldn't eat chocolate or drink red wine, but if you are relying on the "Surely it's better than...?" argument, you might want to ask yourself if you are justifying a particular food or drink when, in truth, you know that there is a better choice that you should make. For example, if you are eating a granola bar instead of a muffin and you tell yourself that because the granola bar is better than the muffin it must be good, then what about eating an apple instead of the granola bar? That's better still. Or if you argue that dark chocolate is better than milk chocolate, how about some dried fruit and a few nuts instead (it's always important to combine the food groups), as they are much better to eat than the dark chocolate?

I am not saying that you shouldn't eat these foods, but please don't fall into the trap of fooling yourself that something is going to be right for you to eat simply because it has an inferior alternative.

Please don't fall into the trap of fooling
yourself that something is going to
be right for you to eat simply because
it has an inferior alternative.

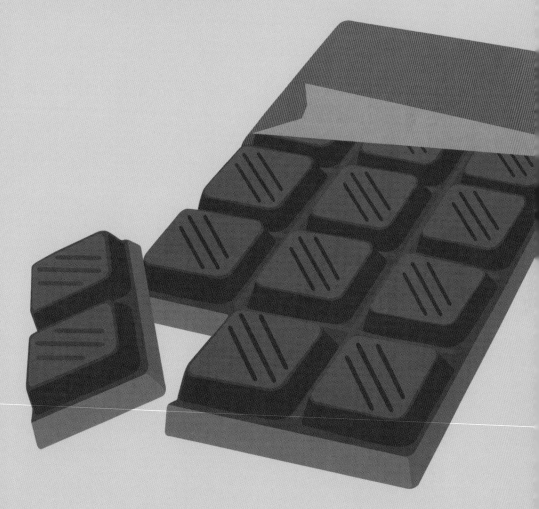

Exercise

In section one we looked at the benefits of exercise on the body's metabolism, and you may remember that in section two I felt uncomfortable with the notion that we should exercise simply to burn off calories. While exercise does, of course, do this, the link isn't as direct as we might want to think it is. In other words, you can't overeat one day and then exercise furiously the next, trusting that your body will use the energy generated by yesterday's food (and only yesterday's food) to fuel your efforts. The body is much cleverer than that, and we really need to have respect for this when deciding upon an exercise routine.

You now know that I favor an eating plan that is both balanced and consistent, and that achieving that balance and consistency through food removes the need to diet and eat in a feast-or-famine cycle. This is equally true of how we should exercise.

A major benefit of regular exercise—in addition to improving our metabolic rate and encouraging efficient blood-glucose management (both key to long-term weight management)—is that it can help to increase our glycogen stores (p.26). This means we can store more glucose in the short-term, rather than converting it into fat for longer-term storage .

To enjoy all the benefits that exercise has to offer, you need to exercise or be active for at least 30 minutes a day, five times a week. That 30 minutes can be divided into smaller chunks of time if it's easier, but 30 minutes is the minimum required amount of time, and ideally you should be aiming for more. However much time you devote to physical activity, the type of exercise you choose has to be considered in the light of two key factors: practicality and enjoyment. Both are vital, or you will start exercising with gusto, life will get in the way, and you will wind down and stop exercising completely.

Practical issues

Whatever you choose to do, whether it's three 10-minute walks every day, or walking the dog for 15 minutes and then boxing for 15 minutes, it must be a routine that is practical and sustainable.

Also under the heading of practicality are a few other qualifying aspects to consider:

1 Affordability
Whether it is a gym membership, fees for a trainer or instructor, clothing, or equipment, in order to be practical it has to be something that you can afford. Not just now, today, but comfortably affordable on your budget for the long term.

2 Geography
Make sure that the gym, swimming pool, or park that you prefer is one that you can get to easily. Wherever your chosen venue, make it as local as possible so that the problem of distance or ease of access isn't going to hamper your regular schedule.

3 Weather
If bad weather is going to interfere with a consistent routine, you may want to consider choosing something that is less reliant upon the weather, or resolve not to let inclement weather deter you.

4 Consistency
The trick here is to engage in physical activity on a consistent basis. Build it into your day and your week by making enough time for it.

Enjoyment
Physical activity, exercise, and sports are all enormously enjoyable, but to ensure that you do something on a consistent basis, you must find something that you enjoy. Whatever that may be, it has to inspire and interest you so that it is not simply a task that has to be undertaken.

So, once you have found something that is practical and enjoyable, please make sure that you enjoy it three or four times a week. Don't be limited to one source of activity: add in walking, swimming, tennis, and anything else to keep it varied and interesting.

The issue of fat clothes

In section two (pp.124–25) we touched on the issue of clothing—fat clothes and thin clothes. I am sure that we all have clothes that fit us better when we are a couple of pounds lighter than usual, and those that we reach for when the opposite is true. Our clothes might have the same size on the labels but the cut of each garment is different, so while one size 12 might be snug, the other is more generous.

Seasoned dieters tend to keep clothes in a variety of sizes and buy smaller clothes along the way to use as an incentive to lose weight again. Having that "little black dress" to fit into is always a useful tool to inspire a healthier lifestyle, because the fit of a close-fitting garment will quickly reveal any weight loss or gain.

Every television show I have worked on that involved weight loss featured a "before" and "after." In the "before" look, the participant is often shown as they first presented themselves, which is always in their own clothes and without the benefit of having been looked after by the hair and makeup department. When it comes to the "after" look, the participant is groomed and styled, which obviously improves their overall appearance (at least for the cameras). However, the underlying question is, will someone who has just lost weight and improved their appearance keep their large trousers, just in case?

Just as the mere existence of diets affords the opportunity for someone to take their eye of the ball for a few days or weeks and gain weight (knowing that they intend to lose it again), I think that knowing that you may have a wardrobe that allows for weight gains and losses actually does the same thing.

My advice about "fat clothes" may seem basic, but it does work. If you are a size 10, but keep a few clothes for when you are feeling a little plump, that's no problem. However, if you are a 10, but keep the size-12 and even the size-14 clothes, just in case, then ditch them, especially the size 14s. In the same way that having a line of credit on your checking account allows you to spend more than you might have, having those larger clothes sitting in your closet might be a contributing factor to repeated weight gain and subsequent loss.

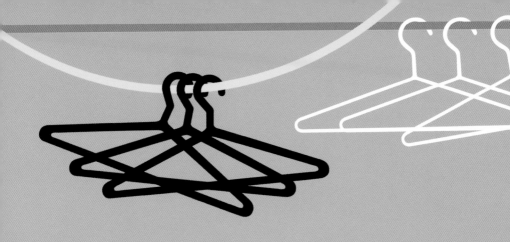

There is nothing to be gained from keeping the larger sizes, so take them all out of your closet and donate them to your local thrift shop today.

If you find that you feel comfortable in your size-10 jeans, but are worried that you might have gained a little weight following a vacation, for example, it's natural to wear the size-12 clothes for a while. But do try on the size 10s and maybe wear them for a couple of hours as a gentle reminder of how they feel and fit compared to how they did a couple of weeks ago. You may wish to remember how you felt in those smaller clothes. Assuming that they made you feel good, feeling uncomfortable in them now as you strain to get into them and wear them for a couple of hours is a great reminder of how you could feel again if they fitted properly, and how you should eat sensibly so that you can feel that way once more.

In the same way that having a line of credit on your checking account allows you to spend more than you might have, having those larger clothes sitting in your closet might be a contributing factor to repeated weight gain and subsequent loss.

Values: what's important to you? There are

countless reasons why we should maintain a healthy weight, but what is most important to us often changes depending on a whole host of influences. When I work with clients who have a history of significant fluctuations in their weight, we often try to pinpoint what weight loss, weight gain, and good health mean to them. We do this by highlighting their own values, which can drive their behavior in one direction or the other. The way we do this involves compiling a list of words that represent something to them, which allows them to understand what motivates them as individuals.

I am sure that if I asked you if you valued your health, the answer would be "yes." However, this straightforward answer immediately raises more problematic questions: Have you had to cut alcohol out completely? Do you have to make time to exercise and have less time to watch TV as a result? Do you have to watch your family eat desserts and not eat them yourself?

The comparison between our finances and weight comes to mind again: When it comes to managing our money, we know that we have to budget in order to make what we earn and what we spend balance out. If we spend too much money on buying, say, a new suit, then we won't be able to pay for the new furnace. If the furnace is more important to us and we value it more than a suit, obviously we would pay for the furnace instead. Our values do change in time, however. The furnace, for example, might be more important than the suit if the weather is cold and your heating keeps breaking down.

So, while we may all pay lip service to wanting to be healthy and slim, do we value television more? Can we really not live without eating dessert every day? I would like you to write down a list of values represented by a single word that will help to establish what is important to you. There is no right or wrong here, so feel free to respond in any way that feels comfortable.

Here are some examples of how we might feel about ourselves, all of which have a positive slant:

- ▸ Successful
- ▸ Accepted
- ▸ Happy
- ▸ Content
- ▸ Vital
- ▸ Powerful
- ▸ Sexy
- ▸ Attractive
- ▸ Recognition
- ▸ Respected
- ▸ Proud
- ▸ Healthy

And some negative ones:

- ▸ Unhealthy
- ▸ Inferior
- ▸ Guilty
- ▸ Rejected
- ▸ Stupid
- ▸ Ashamed
- ▸ Disappointed
- ▸ Regretful
- ▸ Disgusted
- ▸ Frustrated
- ▸ Unattractive
- ▸ Worthless

Ask yourself if these or any other terms represent how you feel about your body, your weight, and exercise. For example, you might think that your body makes you feel proud, which is a positive value. Recognizing this helps you to focus on that feeling and is likely to motivate you to do more things that make you feel proud. Conversely, if you are ashamed of your body, realizing this can motivate you to make changes. There is no right or wrong; this is simply an exercise to help you understand how you feel and make some changes accordingly.

If you do have negative thoughts about your body or weight, this may drive you to consider restrictive dieting in order to get quick results. Please bear in mind that such behavior can compound the issues, as the human body won't respond in the way you want it to in the long run.

Phrases to remove from your life While
we are looking at words and language, let's look at some of the
phrases dieters use, ones that I think are potentially unhelpful.
Listed below are some phrases that I am sure you have heard or
even used yourself. I don't mean to be unsympathetic or sound
overly harsh, but I do think that several of them are unhelpful
to say the least, while others promote overeating, followed by
undereating. Beneath each phrase I offer a reality check or a
solution that accords with my eating plan, and which will help
you to feel liberated from having to think about or mention
such phrases again:

"I have a sweet tooth."
By following my plan, your sugar cravings will reduce so that you
find sweet foods noticeably less desirable.

"Am I allowed ...?"
Yes, you can eat what you like. No food is out of bounds, except for
sugar (see pp.154–55).

"Can I have ...?"
Yes. Why not?

"Work it off in the gym later."
Indulging in sweet or fatty foods and thinking that you can work
them off later perpetuates a desire for these foods, but the most
important point is that as your body has no idea that you are
planning not to store it, the chances are that much of it will
already be stored away by the time you start exercising.

"Make up for it tomorrow."

This keeps you on the "good/bad," "sin/reward" cycle. Furthermore, by the time you really do try to make up for it, the food has already been converted into glycogen and stored away. Lastly, repeatedly indulging upsets your metabolic rate as you eat too much, then too little, then too much again.

"I won't eat tomorrow."

You *will* eat, and your metabolism is far too evolved to fall for this trick. Your body will assume that you are experiencing a famine and try to store food away to make up for the lack.

"Who cares? I can start again tomorrow."

You do care. Or at least you will!

"I've been so good."

There is no "good" and "bad," but staying slim and healthy is the most valuable reward.

"I deserve it."

Of course you do, but you also deserve to be liberated from having to diet constantly.

"You deserve it."

This isn't the most supportive of phrases.

"It will see you through the morning."

You shouldn't expect your food to sustain you so long; it simply has to see you through two and a half hours. This phrase also supports the idea that eating is bad and has to be controlled in a fearful manner.

Final thoughts

Well, there you have it: how NOT to get fat. We have looked at how the body works when it comes to turning food into either energy or fat. We have also examined how we think, feel, and behave and what influences our thoughts, feelings, and behavior when it comes to matters of weight and diet.

Lastly, we have looked at a practical way to eat that directs food to becoming energy rather than allowing it to be stored as fat. I am sure that there are a few people who may have read the last section and thought "Is that it?" The answer to that is a resounding "Yes." If you were hoping for some secret to be revealed, something that only an industry insider like me would know, if you think about it, that's exactly what you have got. The secret is that there is no secret. The vast majority of what we learn about food and weight is always from a diet perspective—in other words, how to lose weight once you have gained it. *How Not To Get Fat* is all about learning how to eat without becoming fat in the first place.

I have been following the method I've outlined in section three for at least a decade, as have countless numbers of my clients. Like them, I can't imagine any other way of eating now. It has become second nature to me. Unlike any diet, my method encourages us to eat, not to abstain from eating. There is no self-control, willpower, or denial required. The most important benefit of my method is that it does not assume that we are greedy, insatiable gluttons who wage a daily battle with food. Rather than extremes, it creates a gentle and manageable level of hunger that allows us to eat rather than starve.

On a practical level my plan will allow you to eat and enjoy food rather than resisting it, which means that you can avoid a life of dieting.

Having come this far, there are a couple of things that I suggest you can do to make life easier for yourself. Firstly, after eating a main course, if you find that you want something sweet, simply go and clean your teeth, rather than battling against it. I find that any sugar cravings, mild though they may be, almost immediately disappear if you follow this advice.

Secondly, remember that consistency is paramount: the way you eat today is the way you will eat next week and next month. Creating that consistency encourages your energy levels to remain constant, and will effectively reassure your body that you are not in famine mode, which can lead to weight gain.

And thirdly, enjoy your food. We live in plentiful times and we are able to eat wonderful food from all over the world. It would be a great shame to deny ourselves the pleasure of eating. Adopting my method allows us to do just that—eat and enjoy.

INDEX

ACKNOWLEDGMENTS

With grateful thanks to Susannah Steel for her patience and good humor, and to everyone at Quadrille, especially Jane O'Shea, Helen Lewis, Clare Lattin, and Mark McGinlay. My special thanks go to my colleagues at The Food Doctor, especially Erika Andersson.